I0693338

INSPIRED
PLANT-BASED PARTIES

Enjoy Food You Crave, Menus, Recipes, Party Themes and Wellness Classes to Slow Aging and Lose Weight

BARBARA BARKER

BALBOA.PRESS

A DIVISION OF HAY HOUSE

The information, ideas, and suggestions in this book are not intended as a substitute for professional medical advice. Before following any suggestions contained in this book, you should consult your personal physician. Neither the author nor the publisher shall be liable or responsible for any loss or damage allegedly arising as a consequence of your use or application of any information or suggestions in this book.

Balboa Press books may be ordered through booksellers or by contacting:

Balboa Press
A Division of Hay House
1663 Liberty Drive
Bloomington, IN 47403
www.balboapress.com
1 (877) 407-4847

Because of the dynamic nature of the Internet, any web addresses or links contained in this book may have changed since publication and may no longer be valid. The views expressed in this work are solely those of the author and do not necessarily reflect the views of the publisher, and the publisher hereby disclaims any responsibility for them.

The author of this book does not dispense medical advice or prescribe the use of any technique as a form of treatment for physical, emotional, or medical problems without the advice of a physician, either directly or indirectly. The intent of the author is only to offer information of a general nature to help you in your quest for emotional and spiritual well-being. In the event you use any of the information in this book for yourself, which is your constitutional right, the author and the publisher assume no responsibility for your actions.

Any people depicted in stock imagery provided by Getty Images are models, and such images are being used for illustrative purposes only.
Certain stock imagery © Getty Images.

Print information available on the last page.

ISBN: 978-1-9822-3430-0 (sc)
ISBN: 978-1-9822-3429-4 (hc)
ISBN: 978-1-9822-3431-7 (e)

Library of Congress Control Number: 2019913007

Balboa Press rev. date: 01/30/2020

Contents

Introduction

I love adapting my traditional family recipes into plant-based inspired elegant fare. I will show you how to do this by offering plant-based party themes and recipes.

Food can bring family and friends together. Every meal can be a time for you to showcase exciting plant- based appetizers, entrees and desserts.

Food can also be used as medicine to create good health. My recipes will help you incorporate "power foods", in other words, plant based options into traditional meals. I offer ancient food wisdom and recent food research in many of the recipes.

Everyone loves desserts, including me. However, I want them to be plant-based, sugar free, salt free, very low fat and gluten free (my niece has Celiac's disease). I also want them to be delicious versions of my grandmother's, mom's and sisters homemade treats: carrot cake, cookies, tiramisu, etc. So I offer adapted dessert recipes.

This book can also be used as a guide for teaching plant-based cooking classes. One appetizer, one entrée, one dessert, one class at a time.

This is more than a plant-based cookbook. It contains classes and information for nurturing your soul and spirit for health and happiness. You will learn how to accomplish your goals.

I am a trained acupressure therapist. As such, I will share with you healing miracles I have learned in thirty years of applied therapy. These lessons teach shortcuts to emotional maturity, which in turn leads to getting along with others.

Awareness is our best tool for our own healing and good health. To prevent illness and live a quality, happy life, be aware of what you are eating. Be aware of how much exercise you get via gardening, stretching, yoga, walking, etc. Make wise food choices. Spend your time and money on buying fruit and vegetables, instead of ingredients which could make you ill.

The latest research and many doctors advise we must follow a plant-based lifestyle to be well. It may even slow aging and help with weight loss.

Acknowledgements

With deep gratitude to my sister, Edith for tasting all my recipes and helping me create some of them.

Dedication

This book is dedicated to my mom, Ethel Rosalyn, to my sisters, Edith Inez and Mary Margaret and to my grandmother Inez.

1

Appetizer Choices

Beverage~

Tropical tarragon iced tea

Appetizer Choices~

No yeast bread with pesto topping

No oil, No cheese, No nuts Pesto

Kale Pesto

Spinach filling

Zucchini Biscuits topped with pesto

Candied Roasted Vegetables

Zucchini Bread

Dessert Choices~

Sweet Potato Cranberry Bread

Cranberry Chutney

Spiced Plum tea sandwich

Beverage

TROPICAL TARRAGON ICED TEA

Ingredients:

¼ cup orange juice

¼ cup pineapple juice

10 drops of liquid stevia or 100% maple syrup*

1 tablespoon lime juice

2 cups tarragon tisane** or tarragon tea***, or 1 tablespoon dried tarragon or 6 sprigs of fresh tarragon

4 cups filtered water (not tap water)

3 black tea bags (try black pomegranate)

Method:
For overnight tea, use an 8 cup capacity pitcher. If using 1 tablespoon dried tarragon, add it to the pitcher with the above ingredients (except the tisane), steep in the refrigerator overnight.

To serve: place a small strainer over an iced tea glass and pour overnight tea into glass, allowing space for ice cubes. Garnish with mint leaves.

*I tablespoon maple syrup

***Three ways to make tarragon tea:**

Method one:
Place 1 *tablespoon* dried tarragon leaves (bottled spice is acceptable) into a tea ball or wrap in cheesecloth and tie into a pouch. Add tea ball or pouch to 2 cups filtered water and refrigerate overnight. Remove tea ball or pouch and add tarragon tea to tropical tea ingredients listed above

Method two
Wrap 6 sprigs of fresh tarragon in cheesecloth and tie into a pouch. Add pouch to 2 cups filtered water and refrigerate overnight. Remove pouch and add tarragon tea to tropical tea ingredients as listed

Method three
**Tarragon tisane: Boil 2 cups filtered water in a small saucepan. Add 1 tablespoon dried tarragon leaves or 6 sprigs of fresh tarragon. Reduce to low heat and simmer 10 minutes. Cool. Using a fine sieve, strain into a large pitcher.

Special note: to make this a fizzy drink: In an iced tea glass half filled with ice cubes, fill ¾ of the glass with tropical tarragon iced tea and fill ¼ of the glass with sparkling water (try lime flavored).

Health benefits of tarragon:
Good for heart health, due to antioxidants, neutralizing free radicals. Treats toothache and water retention. Good for digestion and insomnia. May help protect against the growth of cancer cells.*

*Reference: see Enlightened High Tea Parties book by Barbara Barker.

Find ways you can be a blessing to others every day.

Friendship warms the heart and heals the soul.
Friendship lessens our grief and doubles our joy.

A Friend

Strengthens the heart,
repairs the hurt,
encourages the discovery,
enlightens the mind,
dissolves the pain,
banishes the loneliness,
understands the anxieties,
increases the joy.

Walter Rinder

APPETIZER CHOICES

NO YEAST BREAD WITH PESTO TOPPING

Dry Ingredients:

1 cup flour (any flour you like)

½ teaspoon baking powder (try aluminum free)

¼ teaspoon baking soda

¼ teaspoon salt (optional)*

Wet Ingredients:

½ cup plant based milk (almond milk)

½ tablespoon lemon juice

2 drops liquid stevia or ¼ teaspoon maple syrup

1 ½ tablespoons olive oil

1 tablespoon flaxseed meal dissolved in 3 tablespoons of warm water & let sit 15 to 30 minutes, then stir with a fork until frothy.**

*Salt is optional if using gluten free flour:

Salt keeps bread from tasting flat.

**This is called a flax egg (see chapter 9).

Method: Pre-heat oven to 350 degrees F.

Sift together dry ingredients into a medium mixing bowl. Combine wet ingredients in a small bowl and stir well. Add wet ingredients to dry ingredients and blend well. Spoon batter into an olive oil or Baker's Joy sprayed Bundt pan or 8 inch X 8 inch baking pan/dish. Bake at 350 degrees F for 30 minutes. Insert a toothpick into center of bread; if it comes out clean, your bread is done. Chill completely before cutting with a serrated knife.

Special note:

This bread is a sourdough style bread.

Wrap in plastic wrap and keep refrigerated up to three days. Bread is easier to cut if well chilled.

Place in freezer bag and keep frozen one month.

This bread may be sliced thin for closed sandwiches or cut thick into 2 inch X 2 inch squares as a base for appetizer toppings (Top with pesto recipe below).

Special note: Natural sources of vitamin E include; sunflower seeds almonds and olive oil.

You may add sunflower seeds and/or sliced almonds to this bread for crunch if not allergic to seeds or nuts.

NO OIL, NO CHEESE, NO NUTS PESTO

Ingredients:

4 cups fresh dandelion greens (or 1 cup each fresh leaves of basil, sorrel, parsley, dandelions).

2 cloves peeled garlic

½ cup cooked quinoa or cooked brown rice

2 teaspoons lemon juice

¼ cup warm water

1 teaspoon jarred horseradish

2 teaspoons flaxseed meal

Method:

Process above ingredients in a food processor until smooth. The rice or quinoa makes this a creamy pesto. Keep refrigerated until ready to serve.

Special note: Add seven green olives* (pitted) and three tablespoons olive brine to change the flavor to briny,(salty).

*Try Castelvetrano green olives. They are buttery and briny.

Health benefits of garlic and horseradish: They are natural antibiotics.

Dr. Mercola. Mercola.com

<u>KALE PESTO</u>

Ingredients:

2 cups blanched or sautéed kale leaves*

½ tablespoon lemon or lime juice

¼ cup sliced almonds**

1 clove garlic, peeled

1 tablespoon olive oil or tahini**

¼ cup plant-based shredded cheese**

¼ cup warm water

Optional add ins:

1 teaspoon horseradish (spicier),

1 tablespoon flaxseed meal (firmer),

2 ounces of plant-based cream cheese (creamier).

Method:
Process above ingredients in a food processor to a smooth puree.
Keep refrigerated until ready to serve. Keeps in refrigerator for
2 days. Do not freeze with raw garlic in the pesto.
*Remove stems from leaves

Special note: ** To omit nuts, cheese, cream cheese, oil, and
tahini, add ½ cup cooked brown rice or cooked quinoa Texture
will still be creamy.

***Always eat kale blanched or sautéed (5 minutes), as raw kale
has a harmful effect on the thyroid and kidneys. Raw kale
slows down the thyroid.**

Dr. Oz

Ways to serve kale pesto:

- Mix with hot pasta noodles
- Layer kale pesto on pizza crust instead of tomato sauce, then add vegetables of choice
- Use as a filling inside a quesadilla
- Use as a filling for a tea sandwich
- Use as a spread for an open faced sandwich, then add vegetables of choice.
- Use as a topping for no yeast bread squares
- Serve as a dip for crackers, tortilla chips or pita chips

***Health benefits of kale*:** The leafy cousin of broccoli actually reduces bloating and flatulence. Contains powerful antioxidants, as well as Quercetin. Lowers blood pressure and protects the heart. Cruciferous vegetables contain Vitamin C, Vitamin K, Lutein (eye health) and Beta Carotene. Kale has anti-inflammatory, anti-carcinogen, anti-viral and anti-depressant properties. It may help lower cholesterol.

Healthline.com by K.Gunnars.

Baked kale chips: Wash, rinse, de-stem leaves. Arrange leaves on non-stick parchment paper. Spray with olive oil (or not). Bake at 300 degrees F for 20 minutes.

<u>**SPINACH FILLING**</u>

Ingredients:

1 cup frozen spinach, thawed and squeezed dry

6 ounces tofu* (½ a package) or ¼ cup yogurt**

1 clove garlic, peeled

¼ cup cooked onion, small dice-or-fresh chives,

or 1 teaspoon onion powder

1 teaspoon balsamic vinegar or lemon juice

1 teaspoon each: dried dill, dried parsley or 1 tablespoon vegetable soup mix

2 ounces plant based cream cheese or ½ cup cooked brown rice

Optional add-ins:

½ cup cooked celery (wetter)

1 tablespoon flaxseed meal (firmer)

Method:
Process above ingredients in a food processor until smooth. Makes approximately 2 cups. Keep refrigerated until ready to serve. Serve as a dip.

*Extra firm silken tofu

**Plain, unsweetened plant-based yogurt or unsweetened vanilla plant-based yogurt.

ZUCCHINI BISCUITS

Dry ingredients:

½ cup organic oat flour (store bought or grind organic rolled oats in a food processor to a flour)

1/8 cup millet flour*

½ teaspoon baking powder (aluminum free)

¼ teaspoon baking soda

1/8 teaspoon salt (optional)

1 teaspoon dried parsley**

Wet ingredients:

Half a zucchini grated or 1 carrot grated

2 tablespoons olive oil

1 flax egg (1 tablespoon flaxseed meal dissolved in 3 tablespoons warm water. Let sit 30 minutes and froth with a fork, then add to wet ingredients).

*Use oat flour if you cannot find millet flour. The millet flour makes this a soft biscuit.

**Parsley kills cancer cells. Has antioxidants for liver health.

Foodrevolution.org.

Method: Preheat oven to 350 degrees F.

Sift dry ingredients into a medium mixing bowl. Combine wet ingredients in a small mixing bowl. Add wet ingredients to dry ingredients and combine well. Drop by tablespoon onto a non-stick parchment paper lined baking sheet. Flatten with back of a spoon to ¼ inch thick. Bake at 350 degrees F for 20 minutes. Makes 12 small biscuits. Use as a base for pesto and spreads.

CANDIED ROASTED VEGETABLES

1 pound washed root vegetables*bite size cut

¼ cup 100% maple syrup plus ¼ cup water

2 teaspoons vinegar (balsamic vinegar is sweet)

A pinch of salt and pepper

2 tablespoons olive oil

1 teaspoon dried thyme

Method: Preheat oven to 350 degrees F.

In a non-metallic mixing bowl, combine sauce ingredients and stir well. Add vegetables and stir to evenly coat them. Spread sauced vegetables on a non-stick parchment paper lined baking sheet. Drizzle with 100% maple syrup (or not). Bake at 350 degrees F for 1 hour. Test with paring knife.
*Carrots, Brussel sprouts, or golden beets.

<u>ZUCCHINI BREAD</u>

Dry Ingredients:

1 cup oat flour (store bought or grind organic rolled oats in a food processor to make a flour)

¼ cup rice flour or gluten free baking mix

½ teaspoon baking soda

1 teaspoon Italian seasoning

¼ teaspoon salt (optional)

Wet ingredients:

½ cup grated zucchini

1 flax egg (1 tablespoon flaxseed meal dissolved in 3 tablespoons warm water. Let sit 15 to 30 minutes and froth with a fork).

3 tablespoons almond butter

¼ cup plant-based milk (almond milk)

2 teaspoons vinegar (try balsamic)

Method: Pre heat oven to 350 degrees F.

Sift dry ingredients into a medium mixing bowl. Combine wet ingredients in a small bowl, mix well. Add wet ingredients to dry ingredients and mix well to combine. Pour batter into an olive oil or Baker's Joy sprayed 6 inch X 6 inch baking pan or casserole dish. Bake at 350 degrees F for 40 minutes. Test to see if toothpick inserted in center of bread comes out clean. Cool in the pan. Chill before slicing with a serrated knife. May be sliced thin for a closed sandwich or cut into 2 inch X 2 inch thick squares for topping with pesto, etc.

An Irish Blessing from the 5th Century

May You Have…

enough happiness to keep you sweet

enough trials to keep you strong

enough sorrow to keep you human

enough hope to keep you happy

enough failure to keep you humble

enough success to keep you eager

enough friends to give you comfort

enough wealth to meet your needs

enough enthusiasm to look forward

enough faith to banish depression

enough determination to make each day

better than yesterday.

Author unknown

DESSERT CHOICES

SWEET POTATO CRANBERRY BREAD

Dry Ingredients:

½ cup organic oat flour*

¼ cup organic rolled oats

¼ cup rice flour or gluten free baking mix**

1 teaspoon baking powder (aluminum free)

¼ teaspoon baking soda

¼ teaspoon salt (optional)

¼ teaspoon each cinnamon, ginger, cardamom

Wet Ingredients:

1 cup sweet potato puree or pumpkin puree***

1/3 cup date syrup****

¼ cup lekvar (prune puree)*****

1 tablespoon olive oil

1 teaspoon vanilla extract

2 flax eggs ± (recipe below)

½ cup Craisins, chopped (dried cranberries)

*Store bought or grind organic rolled oats in food processor to flour consistency.

**Kroger brand

***Cooked, peeled and mashed. Canned is acceptable

**** Date syrup: Soak 1 cup pitted dates, in 1 cup warm water 15 minutes. Add to food processor with a cut up orange (including skin) and process to a puree.

*****Lekvar is prune puree. Buy at grocery store or buy baby food prune puree. Lekvar recipe: 2/3 cup pitted prunes (4 ounces) and 3 tablespoons water. Process in food processor to a smooth paste.

± 2 flax eggs: 2 tablespoons flaxseed meal mixed with six tablespoons warm water and stir with a fork until frothy.

Method: Preheat oven to 350 degrees F

Sift dry ingredients into a medium mixing bowl. Combine wet ingredients in a separate medium mixing bowl and stir well to combine. Add wet ingredients to dry ingredients and stir well. Pour batter into an olive oil or Baker's Joy sprayed 8 inch X 8 inch baking pan/dish. Bake at 350 degrees F for 35 minutes. Test with a toothpick to see if done. Chill well before slicing.

Health benefits of prunes and cranberries:

- Prunes create strong bones in your body
- Cranberries prevent urinary tract infections. Cranberries have antioxidants that reduce the level of free radicals, reducing age related damage. Cranberries promote heart health and reduce inflammation and promote healthy digestion. They promote dental health and prevent cancer. *Facty.com*

Think of a moment that brought you joy and focus on that happy place.

Your Hearts Garden

Pull out the weeds of negative thoughts and anger. Plant forgiveness and gentleness. Let others grow in their own way. Be kind. Breathe deep for joy and openness as you release blocked-up emotions that you don't need anymore.

The Herb Companion Magazine.

<u>CRANBERRY CHUTNEY</u>

Ingredients:

8 ounces fresh or frozen cranberries

¼ cup dried apricots, chopped (medium dice)

½ cup orange juice

Method:

In a medium sauce pan, bring above ingredients to a boil, reduce to low heat and simmer 30 minutes.

Off the heat stir in:

1 tablespoon date syrup*

½ tablespoon balsamic vinegar

10 drops of liquid stevia **

Method:

Mash with a potato masher to an almost smooth spread.

Serving suggestion: Spread a thin layer of plant-based cream cheese on a 2 inch X 2 inch piece of firm bread or sweet potato cranberry bread. Top with a small dollop of cranberry chutney. Garnish with parsley leaf or mint leaf.

*Date syrup. (See recipe index)
or
**2 tablespoons 100% maple syrup

<u>SPICED PLUM TEA SANDWICH</u>

Ingredients:

2 large or 4 small pitted dried plums

1 cup prepared cinnamon spice tea

2 tablespoons plant-based cream cheese

5 drops liquid stevia or 1 tablespoon maple syrup

½ teaspoon vanilla extract

1/8 teaspoon ground cinnamon

2 slices of firm bread (cut into 2 inch squares)

1 tablespoon lemon or orange zest (decoration)

Method:

Steep plums and tea 5 minutes. If not softened, cook 15 minutes in spice tea. Mash with a potato masher. In a small bowl mix the cream cheese, 2 teaspoons of prepared spice tea, stevia, cinnamon and vanilla. Mix in the mashed plums. This can also be made in a food processor. Yields ½ cup of filling.

To serve: Spread thinly on bread squares. Sprinkle with lemon or orange zest. This is a special dessert, served on sweet potato cranberry bread.

Special note: Oranges and orange zest help our collagen's elasticity and may prevent wrinkles.

How to Overcome a Health Concern

And Prayer for Good Health

Health issues are created by stress, worrying and thinking the worst about people, places and life experiences. Many healers, including Louise Hay, Barbara Brennan and Brett Bravo believe that our physical problems originate in our emotional body before manifesting as physical illness.

According to the ancient oriental art of balancing life force energy in our body, we can help ourselves by knowing ourselves. If something in the body hurts, it wants to be held. To be healthy, our energy needs to flow freely. Energy that is blocked, due to stress, causes our muscles to tighten. In oriental healing, our body, mind and spirit are balanced by applying our hands to areas of blocked energy in the body. Hands-on-healing, acupressure and Reiki, relax energy blockages that cause pain. Yoga, gardening and deep breathing lower blood pressure and give us a sense of well-being. When energy flows, we receive physical, emotional and spiritual balance.

There are several core components to healing: Reducing stress; Being grateful; Connecting with nature; Reducing isolation; Helping others; Taking care of yourself; Doing gentle physical activity; Being spiritually connected; Eating an organic plant-based diet.

When my late husband was diagnosed as terminal and put on Hospice, my back went out and I couldn't walk. I was in emotional shock. I took acupuncture treatments and did yoga for one and one half years to be able to walk again. I learned I had to believe all things work out for good. I learned that action conquers fear. I prayed. Today I can walk without deformity or pain.

Give the problem to God:

Prayer for Good Health

Lord, you know my health concerns.

Please forgive me of all my sins.

I am sorry for all my sins.

I turn away from sin, back to you Lord.

Please heal all my health concerns,

So I may be of service to you and others.

Amen.

Paraphrased from:

Joyce Meyer Television Ministry

2

Dips, Dressings, Spreads & Bread Choices

Beverage~

Homemade ginger ale

Dips, Dressings, Spreads & Bread choices~

Ranch dip

Tofu sour cream

Tofu mayonnaise

Green olive dip

Beet hummus

Carrot hummus

Sun-dried tomato tofu dip

Pesto ranch dressing

Creamy balsamic vinaigrette

Sweet lemon dressing

Strawberry dressing & salad

Creamy Caesar salad dressing

Reverse aging green herb sauce

Celery spread

Watercress spread

Pesto butter

Arugula pistou

Sun-dried tomato chutney

Golden beet and tahini mousse

Lemon bread

Tofu ricotta bread

Tofu ricotta

Desserts~

Citrus cake

Sweet potato frosting

Strawberry orange jam

Beverage

HOMEMADE GINGER ALE

Ingredients:

1 cup sparkling apple cider (any flavor you like)

1 teaspoon lemon juice

1 teaspoon lime juice

1 teaspoon fresh ginger juice or ginger paste*

8 drops liquid stevia or 1 packet stevia powder or 1 tablespoon 100% maple syrup

Method:
Peel ginger and grate to extract juice. Strain and discard pulp. In a tall glass, combine ginger juice with above ingredients, stir and add ice.

*1/4 teaspoon ginger paste. Buy ginger paste in a squeezable tube in the produce department at the grocery store.

Manufactured by Gourmet Garden.

DIPS, DRESSINGS, SPREADS AND BREADS

<u>RANCH DIP</u>

Ingredients:

1 cup Tofu sour cream*, store bought or my recipe

¼ cup Tofu mayonnaise** (my recipe follows)

1 tablespoons lemon juice

1 clove garlic or ½ teaspoon granulated garlic or ¼ teaspoon garlic salt

¼ cup almond milk

2 tablespoons each dried chives & dried parsley

1 teaspoon Italian seasoning

Method:
Process above ingredients in a food processor until smooth. Keep refrigerated for up to 3 days.

*Replace tofu sour cream with ½ cup plant-based unsweetened yogurt.

**Replace tofu mayonnaise with 4 ounces plant-based cream cheese.

TOFU SOUR CREAM

1 cup Silken extra firm tofu

2 tablespoons olive oil

4 teaspoons lemon juice

¼ teaspoon 100% maple syrup

1/8 teaspoon salt

Method:
Process above ingredients in a food processor until smooth. Cover and chill. Keeps in refrigerator 3 days.

TOFU MAYONNAISE

Ingredients:

½ cup Silken extra firm tofu

1 tablespoon olive oil

1 tablespoon lemon or lime juice

1 teaspoon Dijon mustard

1/8 teaspoon white pepper

Method:
Process above ingredients in a food processor until smooth. Cover and keep refrigerated for 3 days.

<u>GREEN OLIVE DIP</u>

Ingredients:

6 ounces (package) Silken extra firm tofu

1 tablespoon tamari (gluten-free soy sauce)

1 clove garlic (peeled)

¼ cup diced cooked onions

½ cup pitted green olives (about 20 olives. Any green olives you like)

Method:
Process above ingredients in a food processor until smooth. Cover and chill. Keeps in refrigerator 3 days.

To serve: Use as a dip for raw vegetables or cooked potato spears. Dollop on crackers or firm bread. Use as a filling for a tea sandwich.

Special note: This is a salty dip. Limit yourself to 3 vege spears or half a tea sandwich.

What to eat to combat U V rays from the sun:

Strawberries, brazil nuts (limit is 2 per day), tomatoes, green tea (limit 2 cups per day),

Drink 6 glasses of water per day, eat dark chocolate (limit is 1 ounce per day) and watermelon.

BEET HUMMUS

Ingredients:

15 ounce can cannellini beans, rinsed*

1 pound (16 ounces) roasted golden beets** (about 3 medium size beets)

¼ cup tahini or almond butter

2 tablespoons lemon juice

1 tablespoon jarred horseradish

2 cloves peeled garlic

2 tablespoons olive oil

½ teaspoon salt

Method:
Process above ingredients in a food processor until smooth. Cover and chill. Keep refrigerated 3 days.

*Beans are an excellent source of protein, B vitamins and iron. Acceptable to use any bean you like.

**Clean and remove stems from beets. Do not peel. Cut to a large dice. Place onto non-stick parchment paper or non-stick aluminum foil baking sheet and cover with foil. Spray with olive oil. Roast at 400 degrees F for 45 minutes to 1 hour. Test with a paring knife to see if done.

CARROT HUMMUS

Ingredients:

1 cup cooked carrots

¼ cup chopped cooked onions or ½ teaspoon onion powder

1 clove peeled garlic

1 tablespoon olive oil

1 teaspoon curry powder** recipe follows

1 cup cannellini beans (or any bean you like)*

¼ teaspoon turmeric powder

1/8 teaspoon black pepper

Method:
Process above ingredients in a food processor until almost smooth. Cover and keep refrigerated. Serve on bread rounds, raw vegetables or cooked vegetable spears. *Red Kidney beans are very high in fiber.

**Mild Homemade curry powder: 1 tablespoon each: turmeric powder, garlic powder, ginger powder. 1 teaspoon each: ground cloves (powder), coriander powder, cumin powder. Mix in a small bowl and transfer to a shaker bottle.

One hour of walking or doing yoga burns 200 calories.

SUN-DRIED TOMATO TOFU DIP

Ingredients:

4 ounces jarred sun-dried tomatoes in oil or see my recipe for making sun-dried tomatoes.

1 teaspoon Italian seasoning or Herbes de' Provence*

4 ounces silken extra firm tofu

2 ounces plant-based cream cheese

2 cloves peeled garlic

1 tablespoon olive oil

1 tablespoon Kalamata olive brine

¼ teaspoon turmeric powder

1/8 teaspoon black pepper

¼ teaspoon salt

1 plum tomato or ten cherry tomatoes*

Method:
Process above ingredients in a food processor to a smooth puree. Yields 1 cup. Keep refrigerated for up to 3 days.

To serve: Place a small dollop of dip on small bread squares. Garnish with a slice of olive or basil ribbon.

***Special note:** It is acceptable to add fresh tomatoes to this dip if dip is used in one day.

Herbes de Provence:
1 tablespoon each: (dried) Marjoram, Savory, Thyme, Rosemary, Basil, Fennel seeds, Sage and 3 dried food grade lavender buds.

PESTO RANCH DRESSING

Ingredients:

1 cup prepared pesto (jarred or homemade)*

1 cup plant-based buttermilk**or ranch dressing+

Method:
Fold pesto into buttermilk or ranch dressing.

*See recipe index for pesto recipes.

**Plant-based buttermilk recipe: 1 cup almond milk and 1 tablespoon lemon juice. Stir well to combine.

+Quick Ranch dressing: 1 cup plant-based unsweetened yogurt; 2 teaspoons granulated garlic; 1 teaspoon celery salt; 1 tablespoon dried parsley; 1 tablespoon snipped or dried chives.

"Seek the Unique". M. Hinke

To avoid salt, substitute lemon juice, garlic or herbs. All natural foods contain salt. No need to add more salt.

Eat yourself thin book by: C. Carrol

CREAMY BALSAMIC DRESSING

Ingredients:

1 cup silken extra firm tofu

1 tablespoon balsamic vinegar (flavor of choice)

1 tablespoon Dijon mustard

1 clove peeled garlic

1 teaspoon 100% maple syrup or 7 drops liquid stevia

¼ cup water

1/8 teaspoon salt

1/8 teaspoon black pepper

Method:
Process above ingredients in a food processor until smooth. Keep covered and refrigerated up to 3 days.

According to Drs. Lowdog and Oz, spinach, tofu and pumpkin seeds are high in iron and may give you more energy.

Stress stems from being in a hurry, stop hurrying and de-stress.

Dr. Oz.

Complex B vitamins, found in carrots, rolled oats and green leafy vegetables help us metabolize the food we eat, gives good muscle tone, good digestion and healthy nerves.

Eat yourself thin book by: *C. Carrol*

BALSAMIC VINAIGRETTE

Ingredients:

¼ cup unsweetened applesauce

1 teaspoon tamari or soy sauce

1/8 teaspoon cinnamon powder

1 tablespoon balsamic vinegar or lemon juice*

1 teaspoon Dijon mustard

1 tablespoon 100% maple syrup or 7 drops liquid stevia

¼ teaspoon salt

1/8 teaspoon black pepper

1 tablespoon olive oil

Method:
In a small mixing bowl stir above ingredients to blend well. Makes ¼ cup; enough to dress 4 cups of greens.

***Special note:**
This is a sweet dressing. Use lemon juice to temper the sweetness.

Ancient food wisdom: Garlic is for colds and flu. Vinegar is an antifungal, antibacterial and antiviral. Dandelion greens (as in pesto) are a liver cleanse.

SWEET LEMON DRESSING

Ingredients:

2 tablespoons tamari or soy sauce

2 tablespoons lemon juice

2 tablespoons olive oil*

1 tablespoon 100% maple syrup**

Method:
In a small mixing bowl, stir above ingredients until well blended. Makes enough to dress 1 head of lettuce.

*to omit olive oil, substitute Dijon mustard

**To omit maple syrup, substitute 7 drops liquid stevia

Natural sources of Calcium: Dark leafy green vegetables (try dandelions from your back yard), Cabbage, Broccoli, Rolled Oats, Navy Beans, Sunflower Seeds (1 tablespoon per day), Almonds (approximately 7 per day), and Sesame Seeds. Phosphorus works with Calcium for healthy nerves. Natural sources are: nuts, seeds, whole grains, corn and dried fruit. Magnesium, a natural tranquilizer, that also prevents build-up of cholesterol is found in: cooked leafy greens, Kale, Celery, Beets, Apples, Figs, Peaches, Lemons, Almonds, Sunflower Seeds, Sesame Seeds and Brown Rice.

Eat yourself thin book by: C. Carrol

STRAWBERRY DRESSING & SALAD

Ingredients:

1 cup strawberries, cleaned and hulled* or any berries you like

1 tablespoon balsamic vinegar (flavor of choice)

2 tablespoons olive oil

1 tablespoon 100% maple syrup or 10 drops of liquid stevia

*Save a few strawberries for sprinkling on top of salad

Method:
Process above ingredients in a food processor until smooth. Makes enough to dress 1 head of Boston Bibb lettuce.

To serve: Sprinkle quartered strawberries on top of lettuce. Drizzle with dressing. Adapted from the Herb Companion magazine

Optional add-ins:

Red grapes cut in half.
Plant-based shredded cheese.

To grow new brain cells until age ninety and promote longevity: exercise daily, do not smoke, maintain a good weight, get high fiber into your diet, do not consume sugar, eat avocados.

Dr. Perlmutter

CREAMY CAESAR SALAD DRESSING

Ingredients:

½ cup plant-based unsweetened yogurt*

1 teaspoon capers, mashed

1 teaspoon lemon juice

1 teaspoon balsamic vinegar (any flavor)

1 teaspoon Dijon mustard

½ teaspoon Worcestershire (plant-based)

1 clove garlic mashed with a dash of salt

¼ cup plant based parmesan cheese

Method:
Mix ingredients in a small bowl. Keep refrigerated.

*The yogurt replaces oil, egg and mayonnaise.

If you eat 3 cups of bitter greens (such as. dandelions or arugula) and cruciferous vegetables every day, the liver can repair itself. Cruciferous vegetables repair liver cells.

Dr. Oz.

Exercise makes you more sensitive to insulin.

Prevention Magazine.

May you have blue sky days and rainbows.

<u>REVERSE AGING GREEN HERB DRESSING</u>

Ingredients:

2 tablespoons each: fresh basil, chives & parsley

1 teaspoon each dried oregano and thyme (can also use fresh thyme)

1 clove garlic, peeled

2 tablespoons olive oil

2 tablespoons lemon or lime juice

1/8 teaspoon each salt and black pepper

Method:
Process above ingredients in a food process until finely chopped. Serve on pasta, bread or salad greens. Keep refrigerated up to 3 days.

Flax seeds (high in lignans) reduce the risk of Osteoporosis. Acceptable to consume 1 tablespoon per day. Soy and tofu help the bones.

Dr. M. Gregor

"Berries taste great, help you live longer and slow brain aging. Eat a handful a day."

Dr. M. Gregor

Natural sources of Calcium: Chick peas, Tofu, beans, Olive oil, leafy greens and soy milk (limit 1 cup per day). Consuming olive oil and leafy greens together lowers blood pressure.

Prevention Magazine.

CELERY SPREAD

Ingredients:

3 ribs of celery including leaves, cleaned and cut into a medium dice

¾ cup cooked brown rice*

¼ teaspoon celery seeds

1 teaspoon capers

1/8 teaspoon celery salt or tamari or soy sauce

Optional add-ins:

1 tablespoon olive oil, 2 cloves garlic, peeled, 1 teaspoon jarred horseradish.

Method:
Process above ingredients in a food processor to a puree. To make creamier add an additional ¼ cup of rice. Makes 1 ½ cups. Keep refrigerated up to 3 days.

*The rice may be replaced with:

1/3 cup tofu mayonnaise (see recipe index)

1/3 cup tofu sour cream (see recipe index)

4 ounces plant-based cream cheese (store bought)

To serve: Dollop on bread squares, rice cakes or pita chips and garnish with ground caraway seeds. Use as a filling for tortilla spirals (see recipe index). Use as a filling for a closed tea sandwich.

Health benefits of celery: Celery is a super food. It contains apigenin and luteolin, anti-cancer compounds.

Journal of Clinical Biochemistry & Nutrition.

Celery makes breast cancer cells go through cell suicide and can reduce the risk of lung cancer. Takes away pain. Helps with ulcers, diabetes, heart disease, clogged arteries, gout and arthritis.

J. Otto

Health benefits of caraway seeds: Caraway seeds contains fiber and help with digestion. They are one of the oldest cultivated spices (ancient Egyptians); they fight microbes (salmonella) and have antibiotic properties. They increases bone density due to their zinc content. They help with inflammation and mucus build-up. They contain magnesium which promotes good sleep.

Dr. Axe

Health benefits of Purple Tea: Contains red and purple anthocyanins similar to those found in blueberries, raspberries and purple grapes. Red and purple anthocyanins promote weight loss, are anti-aging (rejuvenate skin) and reduces free radicals (cells that can cause degenerative diseases such as diabetes). Betatealtd.com. and infographic.

Health benefits of Cinnamon: Mimics human insulin and controls blood sugar. ¼ teaspoon per day is acceptable.

www.healthline.com

WATERCRESS SPREAD

Ingredients:

½ a bunch of watercress (a handful). Store bought or grow your own (stems removed)

¼ cup plant based unsweetened yogurt*

¼ cup plant-based shredded cheddar cheese

¼ cup plant-based cream cheese

1 teaspoon jarred creamy horseradish

Optional add-ins:

1 tablespoon snipped chives, 1 teaspoon lemon zest, 2 teaspoons lemon juice, 1/8 teaspoon black pepper or ¼ teaspoon garlic powder.

Method:
Process above ingredients in a food processor until smooth. Keep refrigerated.

*Substitute plant-based yogurt with 2 tablespoons either tofu sour cream or tofu mayonnaise. See recipe index for homemade recipes.

To serve: Spread on firm bread of choice. Garnish with a watercress leaf. A great filling for celery boats, baby red potato shells, cherry tomato shells.

Special note: To extend this spread and make it crunchy, add 2 ribs of minced celery. Pulse in food processor to mince). Makes 1 cup of spread.

To make Watercress spiral tea sandwiches: In a food processor combine 1 bunch of watercress, ¼ cup plant-based margarine,

1 clove of garlic. Process to a smooth puree. Keep refrigerated. Using a rolling pin, roll a slice of bread to a 5 inch square. Spread a thin layer of watercress margarine mixture on bread slice and roll up jellyroll fashion. Refrigerate 1 hour to chill. To serve, slice each bread roll into 1 inch spirals. Allow one bread roll (5 spirals) for each guest.

Health benefits of watercress: Watercress is the new kale. A member of the mustard family, watercress contains manganese, folate, carotene, more vitamin C than an orange, more calcium than a glass of milk, prevents strokes and is an anti-depressant. Watercress contains lutein which improves eyesight, heart health, thyroid function, brain cognition, prevents breast and colon cancer and boosts immunity. *Prevention Magazine.*

Before you say something ask yourself:

the truth test: is it true?

the goodness test: is it good?

the useful test: is it useful to you and me?

Socrates

PESTO BUTTER

Ingredients:

2 cups fresh mixed herbs (dandelions, sorrel, lettuce, purslane, basil, spinach, parsley, thyme, or any leafy herbs you like, even nasturtium leaves).

1 teaspoon lemon juice

1 clove peeled garlic

2 tablespoons plant-based margarine

2 tablespoons plant-based cream cheese

A pinch each of salt and pepper

1 tablespoon of olive brine

Method:
Process above ingredients in a food processor to a smooth puree. Yields 1 cup.

To serve: Spread a thin layer of pesto butter on any bread you like. Cut bread into 1 inch squares. Garnish with an olive slice and a lettuce leaf ribbon

Health benefits of Dandelions: Promotes a healthy liver; helps memory; has anti-aging properties; is good for the bones; acts as a diuretic; has anti-cancer (lutealin) properties; reduces inflammation. Is In the daisy and ragweed family.

Healthlinenutrition.com

ARUGULA PISTOU

Ingredients:

3 to 4 cups arugula leaves

1 tablespoon olive oil

2 tablespoons tofu sour cream, store bought *

2 tablespoons warm water

1 clove peeled garlic

Method:
Process above ingredients in a food processor to a smooth puree.
Optional add-ins: 4 sprigs purslane or 8 dandelion leaves.

Pistou is a green sauce from the south of France made without cheese and without nuts.

Pesto is a green sauce from Italy that contains both cheese and nuts.

*For homemade recipe, see recipe index.

To serve: Mix with hot pasta or vegetable noodles. Spread on rice cakes or small squares of firm bread. Use as a filling for baby red potato shells, celery boats or cherry tomato shells. Use as a dip for pita bread.

Italy's blue zones (where many people live to age 100) have followed a plant-based diet for centuries.

Miyoko Schinner

<u>SUN-DRIED TOMATO CHUTNEY</u>

Ingredients:

1 tablespoon olive oil

½ teaspoon Dijon mustard

2 tablespoons chopped onions

2 cups chopped tomatoes

a pinch of salt

1 tablespoon 100% maple syrup

¼ teaspoon powdered ginger

Method:
In a large sauté pan, over medium heat, sauté above ingredients for 5 minutes. Reduce to low heat and simmer 30 minutes. Stir. Let cool in the pan. Makes 1 cup

To serve: Spoon 1 tablespoon over cooked rice or cooked quinoa. Use as a topping for pizza crust of choice, top with vegetables and plant-based cheese. Heat in oven at 350 degrees F for 10 minutes.

Four Core Virtues for a Long-Lasting Relationship~

Honesty (trust). Compromise (adapt),

Patience and Giving (Love and insight).

Tibetan Monks.

GOLDEN BEET AND TAHINI MOUSSE

Ingredients:

1 tablespoon tahini (sesame seed paste)

¼ cup plant-based cream cheese

¾ cup golden beets cooked, including skin

1 tablespoon lemon juice

1 tablespoon pomegranate juice*

1 packet stevia powder or 1 tsp. maple syrup

1 tablespoon date syrup (see recipe index)

¾ teaspoon curry, ginger, garlic mix**

Method:
Process above ingredients in a food processor until smooth. Keep refrigerated. Spread on bread squares. Garnish with a beet slice matchstick.

*Pomegranate sour sauce may be substituted.

**¼ teaspoon each: curry powder, garlic powder and ginger powder. Mix well.

Health benefits of beets: They contain nitric oxide (widens blood vessels) for increased energy and stamina. They contain Vitamins C and B, potassium, fiber, manganese and folate. They lower blood pressure and fight inflammation.

Organicfacts.net.

LEMON BREAD

Dry Ingredients:

½ cup oat flour (store bought or grind rolled oats)

1 teaspoon baking powder

¼ cup organic rolled oats

¼ cup rice flour or baking mix like Bisquick

¼ teaspoon salt (optional)

Wet Ingredients:

½ cup plant-based yogurt, plain or vanilla flavor

½ teaspoon vanilla extract

2 tablespoons maple syrup or date syrup*

2 flax eggs (dissolve 2 tablespoons flaxseed meal in ¼ cup warm water, let stand 30 minutes)

Zest and juice of 1 lemon (about 2 tablespoons)**

1 tablespoon olive oil

2 tablespoons prune puree (see recipe index)

Method: Pre-heat oven to 350 degrees F.

Sift dry ingredients into a medium mixing bowl. Combine wet ingredients in a small mixing bowl. Add wet ingredients to dry ingredients and mix well. Spray a 9 inch X 9 inch glass baking dish with olive oil or Baker's Joy. Pour batter into sprayed dish. Bake at 350 degrees F for 30 minutes. Insert a toothpick into center of bread/cake. If it comes out clean, bread/cake is done.

Special note: This bread/cake is very mild and can be served as a bread for savory toppings or as a cake for sweet toppings. A

9 inch X 9 inch baking dish yields a ½ inch tall bread, suitable as a base for savory toppings (an excellent base for open-faced cucumber tea sandwiches). An 8 inch X 8 inch baking dish yields a 1 inch tall cake suitable for frosting or sweet toppings.

*Do not use stevia as a sweetener in this recipe as it creates a bitter, metallic taste with the lemon. See recipe index for date syrup recipe.

**Acceptable to use lime zest and 2 tablespoons lime juice instead of lemon. Lime juice is sweeter than lemon juice.

Health benefits of lemons and limes (including the zest): They are a good source of vitamin C and prevent kidney stones. They support heart health and protect against anemia. They may reduce cancer risk and improve digestion. They help your immune system. They contain collagen, which may delay skin aging and tightens skin. May lower blood pressure and risk of stroke. Contains potassium which helps the nervous system. Powerful anti-viral and anti-inflammatory.

HealthfitnessRevolution.org.

TOFU RICOTTA BREAD

Dry Ingredients:

¾ cup flour: ¼ cup each oat, rice and quinoa flour

1 teaspoon baking powder

1/8 teaspoon salt

Wet Ingredients:

¾ cup homemade tofu ricotta, see recipe index

10 drops of liquid stevia

2 flax eggs (dissolve 2 tablespoons flaxseed meal in 6 tablespoons warm water. Let stand 30 minutes)

1 teaspoon vanilla extract

1 tablespoon olive oil

Method: Pre-heat oven to 350 degrees F.

Sift dry ingredients into a medium mixing bowl. Mix wet ingredients in a small mixing bowl. Add wet ingredients to dry ingredients and mix well. Spray an 8 inch X 8 inch baking dish with olive oil or Baker's Joy. Spoon batter into a baking dish. Bake at 350 degrees F for 30 minutes. Cool or refrigerate before cutting.

Special note: This is a flat-bread like, a focaccia bread, and may be served as sweet or savory.

<u>HOMEMADE TOFU RICOTTA*</u>

Ingredients:

6 ounces silken extra firm tofu

½ cup sliced almonds

1/8 cup nutritional yeast, buy at health food store

1½ tablespoons olive oil

1/8 teaspoon each salt and black pepper

Method:
Process above ingredients in a food processor, until smooth. Keep refrigerated or freeze.

*You may purchase plant-based ricotta cheese at a health food store. Manufacturer: Tofutti better ricotta cheese.

Olive oil spray: In a glass or plastic spray bottle add ¼ cup olive oil. Use as a spray for coating baking dishes or sauté pans. Add ¼ cup water to the oil if you are limiting oil in your diet.

Protein sources:

To get more plant-based protein in your diet, eat ½ cup beans or legumes (lentils, peas etc.) 3 times per day for adequate protein.

Dr. Mc Dougall.

Foods that boost metabolism: Cinnamon, lemon zest, cumin, garlic, tahini, mint, pomegranate, parsley, cilantro.

Dr. Oz

DESSERT

<u>CITRUS CAKE</u>

Dry Ingredients:

  1 cup flour*

  1 teaspoon baking powder (aluminum free)

  ¼ teaspoon salt (optional)**

Wet Ingredients:

  2 flax eggs (2 tablespoons flax seed meal dissolved in ¼ cup water. Let stand 30 minutes)

  2 tablespoons date syrup (see recipe index)

  2 tablespoons 100% maple syrup***

  2 tablespoons olive oil

  1/8 cup orange juice

  1/8 cup lemon or lime juice

  1 tablespoon citrus zest~ orange, lemon or lime

  1/8 cup plant based yogurt, vanilla or plain flavor

  1 teaspoon vanilla extract

  ½ teaspoon almond extract

Stir-ins:

  ½ cup blueberries or any diced fruit you like. Dried blueberries and dried fruit are acceptable.

Method: Pre-heat oven to 325 degrees F

Sift dry ingredients into a medium mixing bowl. Add fruit and stir to coat, so fruit does not sink to bottom of the cake. Combine wet ingredients in a small mixing bowl. Add wet ingredients to dry ingredients and mix well. Spray an 8 inch X 8 inch baking dish (Corning-ware works well for baking) with olive oil spray. Pour batter into a baking dish, smooth the top and bake at 325 degrees F for 25 minutes, until a toothpick inserted in the middle comes out clean. This cake is a tender crumb and is good with frosting, fresh fruit, jam or as a base for English trifle or tiramisu.

*Try a mixture of ¼ cup each oat flour, quinoa flour, whole wheat pastry flour and Bisquick.

**Salt adds flavor, lightens gluten structure, adds strength to the dough, and balances sweetness. If you are restricting salt, you may omit it without changing texture or flavor.

***To omit maple syrup, increase date syrup to 4 tablespoons. Do not add stevia to baked goods containing citrus as the stevia will create a bitter, metallic flavor.

Passions

Things you love to do. These are your spiritual gifts. See how you can use these gifts to help others. Live your passions. *Paraphrased from James Van Prague)*

SWEET POTATO FROSTING

Ingredients:

2 cups cooked, peeled gold sweet potatoes*

10 drops of liquid stevia**

1 teaspoon vanilla extract

¼ cup plant-based yogurt, plain or vanilla flavor

Method:
Process above ingredients in a food processor, until smooth. If mixture seems dry, add 1/8 cup water or yogurt. Makes enough to frost one cake.

*Gold or Hanna sweet potatoes have a tan skin and white flesh. To roast, wrap in aluminum foil and bake in a pre-heated 400 degree F oven, 1 hour. Test with a paring knife to see if done. Let cool or keep refrigerated. Peel and cut to a large dice before adding to food processor. 1 sweet potato yields 1 cup.

**Substitute light color 100% maple syrup for stevia.

To serve: This frosting has the consistency of a cream cheese frosting. Suitable for carrot cake or any cake you like. Excellent as a topping for fresh fruit or baked fruit. This frosting may also be used as a filling for English trifle or tiramisu. My sister freezes this and I call it ice cream (also good on cake).

STRAWBERRY ORANGE JAM

Ingredients:

1 pound of strawberries* (16 ounces), rinsed, hulled and quartered (approximately 20 strawberries)

1 apple (any variety you like), washed, cored and cut to a small dice

2 tablespoons orange, lemon or lime juice

¼ cup orange or apple juice

½ teaspoon cornstarch dissolved in 2 tablespoons orange or apple juice

1 tablespoon 100% maple syrup or date syrup

Method:

In a medium-sized saucepan cook fruit and juices (first 4 ingredients) over medium heat, uncovered for 15 minutes. In a small bowl dissolve cornstarch in the orange or apple juice. Add to the cooked fruit. Bring to a boil and cook 5 minutes, stirring frequently. Remove from heat. Mash jam with a potato masher. Add sweetener. Stir well. Cool 15 minutes. Makes 2 cups. Keep refrigerated up to 3 days. Chill 2 hours before serving.

To test consistency, put a spoonful of cooked jam on a plate that has been chilled in the freezer 20 minutes. Whatever the thickness of the jam is on the plate will be the consistency of the finished product.

How To Slow Aging Class

Secrets Of Having More Energy

And Quick Pick-Me-Ups

What causes aging? Stress ages us. Damage to the immune system, from free radicals,* ages us. Poor nutrition, alcohol and smoking cause free radicals to multiply and damage cells. Aging happens when there are more free radicals than anti-oxidants.

What slows aging? Anti-oxidants.

The richest food sources of anti-oxidants are: berries, seeds, fruit and vegetables. Specifically, garlic, onions, cruciferous vegetables, Brazil nuts, pumpkin seeds and flaxseed meal.

Fruit and vegetables high in Vitamin C help prevent wrinkles: citrus, pineapple, papaya, strawberries, bell peppers.

Drinking a mixture of cucumber and water can help with bags under the eyes.

The herb rosemary can help with dark circles under the eyes.

The following are herbs for youthful skin: cinnamon, cumin, curry powder, thyme, oregano, turmeric, sage and rosemary.

Additional anti-aging foods include: 2 cups of green tea per day, cooked tomatoes and Vitamin A rich foods, such as apricots, cantaloupe, cooked kale, and sweet potatoes.

Lentils, cocoa powder and quinoa are anti-oxidant rich foods.
Dr. Oz, Dr. Weil, Dr. Yung, Dr. N. Naeem.

*Free radicals are molecules in cells with an odd number of electrons that need to take an electron from our DNA, protein cells or immune cells. Anti-oxidants can give an electron to a free radical, neutralize them, ending the electron stealing and cell damage.

Secrets of having more energy:

Tibetan monks advise there are 4 types of energy: Physical, mental, emotional and spiritual. To have more physical energy, exercise and eat small meals, because big meals drain energy.

Get enough omega three fatty acids: Quinoa, olives, flaxseed meal and avocados.

Get enough iron (beans), Vitamins C, B-12, D-3 and a multi-vitamin.

Practice deep breathing and sleep 8 hours per night.
To have more mental energy: Drink 8 glasses of water per day and exercise your brain.

For emotional energy: avoid critical, complaining people. Make a gratitude list daily.

For spiritual energy: find out what gives your life meaning. Know your purpose. Pray. Help and forgive others.

Dr. Andrew Weil advises the following to have more energy and increase immunity: avoid animal protein and sugar. Add 1 teaspoon of olive oil per day to your diet. Eat fruit, vegetables and a moderate amount of grains. Eat ginger, garlic, turmeric, Vitamin C rich foods and almond milk. To double your energy: eat less, exercise in sunlight, do yoga, laugh, dance and rest.

Quick pick-me-ups:

According to Dr. Oz and Dr. Weil: Parsley (pesto or juice) will give you energy all day long. Eat apples and drink water. Rub your ear lobes. Laugh out loud. Breathe deeply. Take a shower.

Aromatherapy: Peppermint, Spearmint, pine and eucalyptus essential oils energize you.

Try new things. Take a new route to work. Take a nap. Exercise in sunshine (increases serotonin for a good mood). Read a book or learn a new language.

3

Brunch Menu

Beverages~

Cranberry fizz mock tail

Cranberry fizz punch

Brunch~

Baked fruit parfaits

Garden spirals

Tangy sweet cranberry spirals

Strawberry salad

Marinated Vegetables

Dessert~

Chocolate chip sweet potato cookies or cake

BEVERAGES

CRANBERRY FIZZ MOCKTAIL

Ingredients:

¾ cup sparkling cranberry apple juice

¼ cup cranberry juice

Method:
In a tall glass, filled with ice, combine above ingredients. Stir. Garnish with a sprig of mint.

CRANBERRY FIZZ PUNCH

Ingredients:

1 cup cranberry juice (unsweetened)

1 cup pomegranate juice

¼ cup 100% maple syrup

1 tablespoon lime juice

2 cups sparkling cranberry juice

2 cups filtered water (not tap water)

Method: Mix above ingredients in an 8 cup capacity pitcher. Serve over ice. Yields 8 servings.

BRUNCH

<u>BAKED FRUIT PARFAITS</u>

Ingredients for the baked fruit:

1 cup organic rolled oats

1 apple, cored and cut to a medium dice

6 strawberries, hulled and cut into fourths

1 cup blueberries, fresh or frozen

2 cups water or fruit juice of choice

1 teaspoon vanilla extract

1 teaspoon cinnamon

1 cup applesauce, unsweetened

2 packets powdered stevia

Method: Pre-heat oven to 350 degrees F

Using a 9 inch X 13 inch or 10 inch X 10 inch baking dish, sprayed with olive oil, layer ½ cup rolled oats on bottom of dish. Sprinkle with one packet of stevia. Layer fruit over oats in order shown. Spread applesauce over berries. Top with ½ cup rolled oats. Mix vanilla with water or fruit juice and pour over fruit casserole. Sprinkle stevia and cinnamon over oats. Put baking dish on a baking sheet to catch spills. Bake at 350 degrees F for 45 minutes. Makes 8 servings. Keep refrigerated. A healthy breakfast.

Ingredients for parfaits:

Soft cookies or cake of choice

1 carton plant-based vanilla yogurt six ounce

Baked fruit from recipe above

Shelled sunflower or pumpkin seeds

Method:

In a fancy stemmed glass, layer ½ cookie or a small piece of cake in the bottom of the glass. Spoon one tablespoon of yogurt over the cookie. Spoon 2 tablespoons of baked fruit over the yogurt. Spoon one tablespoon of yogurt over baked fruit. Crumble cookie or cake over yogurt. Top with a sprinkle of seeds. Makes one parfait.

Health benefits of cranberries: A super-food, 1 cup contains 46 calories. An anti-oxidant rich food, with more anti-oxidants than blueberries and green tea. May help to prevent cancer or reduce the spread of cancer cells *(Prevention Magazine)*. Boosts the immune system. May help to decrease blood pressure. Reduces arthritis inflammation. Helps with digestion and ulcers. Lowers risk of urinary tract infections. Prevents plaque build-up on blood vessels and teeth. Helps keep arteries clear. A great source of resveratrol, which may slow the sprouting of blood vessels that help tumors grow).

Medical news today.com

GARDEN SPIRALS

Ingredients:

2 ounces plant-based cream cheese

½ cup cooked brown rice

1 cooked carrot, small dice

10 basil leaves, chopped

1 clove minced garlic

1 tablespoon cooked bell peppers, small dice

1 cup cooked green beans, small dice

1 celery rib, small dice

¼ teaspoon garlic salt

1 package flour tortillas

Method:
Mix above ingredients (except tortillas) by hand in a medium mixing bowl. Keep refrigerated. Makes 1½ cups. Spread a thin layer of filling on entire tortilla and roll jellyroll fashion. Place on plate seam side down, cover & chill 1 hour before slicing. Cut into 1 inch spirals to serve. Be creative: use chopped olives, artichoke hearts, water chestnuts, spinach, roasted red bell peppers, chives, green peas. Make lots of spirals; as my sister says "I could eat these all day".

TANGY SWEET CRANBERRY SPIRALS

Ingredients:

4 ounces plant-based cream cheese

½ cup cooked brown rice

½ cup chopped Craisins (dried cranberries)*

1 celery rib, small dice**

7 chives snipped with scissors

1 package flour tortillas

Method:
Mix above ingredients (except tortillas) by hand in a medium mixing bowl. Spoon a thin layer over entire tortilla and roll jellyroll fashion, seam side down. Cover with plastic wrap and chill 2 hours or overnight. Makes about four tortilla rolls. Cut each tortilla roll into one inch pieces and plate cut side showing the spiral. These can be served as a savory or as a dessert.

*Acceptable to substitute any dried chopped fruit you like. Try dried blueberries.

**Add more celery to extend the amount of the filling.

Special note: Mixing this in a food processor makes a watery filling. You may chop the celery or Craisins in the food processor, then add them to the filling and mix by hand.

STRAWBERRY SALAD~ See page 35

MARINATED VEGETABLES*

Ingredients:

1 unpeeled cucumber, washed & cut into coins*

1 cup cauliflower florets*

2 tablespoons tamari or soy sauce

2 cloves of garlic, peeled and minced

1 scallion, diced or 8 chives snipped with scissors

1 teaspoon vinegar (any vinegar you like)

¼ cup water

1 teaspoon 100% maple syrup or 1 packet stevia

1/8 teaspoon each salt and pepper

Method:
In a lidded non-metallic container, marinate above ingredients. Ready to serve after 1 hour. Keeps in refrigerator 3 days. Acceptable to marinate radishes. *Not recommended for broccoli or carrots.
Adapted from my family's recipe

DESSERT

<u>CHOCOLATE CHIP SWEET POTATO COOKIES OR CAKE</u>

Dry Ingredients:

1½ cups flour

½ cup organic rolled oats or granola**

1 teaspoon baking powder

1 teaspoon baking soda

1 teaspoon cinnamon

½ teaspoon salt

1 cup chocolate chips (Lilly's are sugar free)

Wet Ingredients:

2 tablespoons olive oil

2 tablespoons prune puree*

2 tablespoons date syrup*

1 flax egg*

1 teaspoon vanilla extract

1½ cups sweet potatoes, cooked, peeled & mashed (acceptable to use canned)

½ cup plant-based milk + 1 tablespoon lime juice

Method: Pre-heat oven to 375 degrees F

Sift dry ingredients into a medium mixing bowl. In a separate medium bowl combine wet ingredients and stir well. Add wet ingredients to dry ingredients and blend well. On a non-stick parchment paper lined baking sheet, drop dough by tablespoon, sprinkle with rolled oats and flatten to ½ inch thickness. Bake at 375 degrees F for 15 minutes. This is a soft cookie. Makes two dozen.

Method to make as a cake:

Spray a 10 inch X 10 inch baking dish with olive oil spray or Baker's Joy. Spoon dough into a baking dish and sprinkle with rolled oats or granola. Bake at 375 degrees F for 20 minutes, until a toothpick inserted in the middle comes out clean.

*See recipe index

**Add ¼ cup rolled oats or granola for sprinkling cookies or cake before baking.

Chocolate, cranberries, strawberries, pomegranates, black tea and green tea increase polyphenols for clear arteries.

Prevention Magazine

A lady who lived to 114 years gave her secret for longevity….she ate a sweet potato every day.

Life is uncertain…eat dessert first.
Ernestine Ulmer

Wisdom Insights and How to be Happy Class

Wisdom is defined as good judgement. Wisdom is also defined as doing today what will give you a good outcome tomorrow. *(Paraphrased from Joyce Meyer ministries).* According to the Dalai Lama XIV, (paraphrased), wisdom is listening to others and trying to understand others. Encourage others with kind words.

So, how do we get wisdom? Think before you act. Act on your values. Learn from your mistakes. Be humble. Inspire others. Don't complain. Say positive things. Look for the silver lining in situations. What was the good thing I learned in this situation? Look your best, be your best, act your best. Learn the best way to eat for health and make small consistent changes.

To be your best, you must be well. If you don't feel well, you won't act optimally. Here are dietary concepts that will help you feel well and be your best: Eat until 80% full. Eat small portions. Eat slowly. Eat fruit when craving sugar. To heal ourselves and keep our health, eat a plant-based diet (fights off infection). Eat more fiber (there is no fiber in sugar, white flour or alcohol). High fiber foods (about 4 grams of fiber in ½ cup) include: artichokes, spinach, berries, vegetables, prunes, and green peas. Sweeten food with blueberries.

We only get one body….take care of it.

How to be happy: Happiness is an emotion.

List that for which you are grateful. This will lift your mood. Say positive things about yourself and others. Say hopeful, healing words and positive affirmations. Keep your promises to others. Be mindful of the Karma you are creating. Be kind. Appreciate others. When I am appreciated, I am calm and happy. When

I am criticized, I am anxious and grieved (close to tears). Happiness means taking good care of yourself.

Incorporate the following foods into your diet for a better mood: Lentils, beets, avocados, oranges, spinach, matcha green tea*, Brazil nuts (1 per day), pumpkin seeds, dark green leafy vegetables, blueberries and chocolate (boost serotonin and folate). Brazil nuts, mushrooms and lentils boost selenium for increased energy and decreased anxiety. Flaxseeds, chia seeds, olives, avocados and quinoa may boost omega 3 fatty acids for healthy brain function and to fight depression. De-stress and sleep better with magnesium rich foods, such as legumes, leafy greens, nuts and tofu. Eat foods with Vitamin B-6 (for serotonin uptake), such as carrots, sweet potatoes, green peas and lentils. Vitamins C, D and sunshine lessen anger, confusion and depression. Zinc (for better memory), is found in legumes, seeds, nuts and whole grains. De-cluttering your space and talking with friends reduces stress. Acts of kindness make us feel better about ourselves. Be kind to everyone, they could be an angel.

*See my recipe for matcha green tea cookies

RULES FOR HAPPINESS

Something to do...........................

Someone to Love........................

Something to Hope for..................

Immanuel Kant

There is always something

we can succeed at.

As long as there is Life,

there is Hope.

Steven Hawking

4

Lite Lunch Menu

Beverage~

Mock Champagne

Entrée~

Pasta Vegetable salad with rosemary tisane

Kale chips

Dessert~

Sweet potato almond tea bread with jam

BEVERAGE

<u>MOCK</u> <u>CHAMPAGNE</u>

Ingredients:

¼ cup pomegranate juice, chilled

1 tablespoon 100% maple syrup*

1 teaspoon lime juice

½ cup bottled water (not tap water)

½ cup sparkling ICE brand flavored water, grapefruit flavor, chilled or grapefruit juice, chilled

¼ cup orange or cranberry juice, chilled

2 cups ginger ale, chilled

Method:
Combine above ingredients in a 4 cup pitcher. Stir to combine. Serve in a champagne glass or wine glass. Do not add ice. Yields about 3 cups.

*May substitute 7 drops liquid stevia

ENTRÉE

PASTA VEGETABLE SALAD WITH ROSEMARY TISANE

Ingredients:

8 ounces (half a pound) cooked pasta of choice*

1 cup cooked celery, small dice

1 cup cooked broccoli florets

Vinaigrette of choice (try creamy balsamic)

Method:
Cook the pasta in water or rosemary tisane *** until al dente. Cool and add to a large mixing bowl. Steam celery and broccoli and add to pasta bowl. Toss with vinaigrette of choice (see recipes for sweet lemon dressing or pesto ranch). Keep refrigerated. You may add pumpkin seeds and any variety of vegetables. *Rotini or penne style pasta works better than thin pasta.

Rosemary tisane: In a large saucepan, add 4 cups of water and 6 sprigs of fresh rosemary (rinsed). Bring to a boil, reduce heat to low and simmer 10 minutes. Strain into a pasta pot, (discard rosemary) add pasta and cook pasta to al dente. You may tie rosemary in a cheesecloth bag to avoid having to strain the tisane. You may also cook rice in rosemary tisane.

KALE CHIPS: See page 9 and recipe index

DESSERT

SWEET POTATO ALMOND TEA BREAD

Dry Ingredients:

1 cup flour

¼ cup organic rolled oats + ¼ cup for sprinkling on bread before baking

1¼ teaspoon baking powder

¼ teaspoon baking soda

1/8 teaspoon salt

¼ teaspoon cinnamon

¼ teaspoon pumpkin pie spice

Wet Ingredients:

2/3 cup cooked mashed sweet potatoes, (acceptable to use canned)

¼ cup plant based almond milk

2 tablespoons olive oil or almond butter

1 flax egg (see recipe index)

1 tablespoon 100% maple syrup (optional)

Stir ins: ¼ cup sliced almonds

Method: Pre-heat oven to 350 degrees F

In a medium mixing bowl sift together dry ingredients. In a small mixing bowl combine wet ingredients and stir well. Add wet ingredients to dry ingredients and stir to blend well. This is a wet sticky dough. Spoon batter into a bundt pan sprayed with olive oil or Baker's Joy (acceptable to use a 9 inch X 5 inch loaf pan (sprayed) or 8 inch X 8 inch baking dish, sprayed. Sprinkle top of batter with ¼ cup rolled oats. Bake at 350 degrees F for 40 minutes (may require 50 minutes in the loaf pan). Completely baked when a toothpick inserted in the middle comes out clean. Slice with a serrated knife when well chilled to avoid crumbled slices.

To Serve:
Serve topped with jam (see strawberry orange jam, Chapter 2) or sweet potato frosting (Chapter 2) or top with fresh or cooked fruit.

Health benefits of almonds: Rich in anti- oxidants to promote healthy skin and prevent signs of aging. A good source of vitamin E (anti-inflammatory). Contains healthy fats that help us absorb vitamins and nutrients from our food to give us energy. Regulates blood sugar levels and helps with insulin resistance. Helps to maintain a healthy weight, due to high fiber. Can reduce inflammation in the brain. Can reduce cholesterol and prevent heart disease. Helps the immune system. Promotes healthy digestion. Anti-oxidants can prevent cancer, by free radical reduction.

10FAQHealth.com

How to Manifest ~

Having Your Dreams Come True

Manifesting your dreams is a multi-faceted process. It involves having a clear and concise vision of what you want in your life. You cannot manifest by focusing on the negative thoughts of: I don't want this, that or the other; or I hate this, that or the other.

To manifest a dream, your ideas, thoughts affirmations and actions must match your dream. Whatever you focus on and believe, becomes real for you. Saying positive affirmations can change your future. My all-encompassing affirmation attracts good people and good fortune into your life. Try it and see if you feel better about what's coming to you:

Affirmation

I am surrounded by healthy, wealthy, wise, kind people who have my best interests at heart, and who generously support all my work and all my creative endeavors.

You can also change your future by changing any negative affirmations. Change: *I am so in debt,* to affirm: *I am now free of debt.* Change: *I am not well,* to affirm: *I am disease free because my body wants to heal.* Change: *I'll never get a job,* to affirm: *Good people will give me a great job.* Change: *I don't have enough,* to affirm: *I have plenty to meet my needs and enough to give away.*

Take an inventory of all the good things you have in your life now and how others have helped you. Be thankful for what's going right in your life. Ask the universe to show you how you can help others. Don't be negative, and don't be an unhappy victim. Dress beautifully every day. If you feel good, you act good. Be inspired to connect your actions with your dreams. Instead of doubting the outcomes, imagine the great possibilities. Act as if you already have what you want. Say: this is true for me. Don't say: I can have what I want, *after* this or that happens.

According to Edgar Cayce (renowned psychic), prepare a written inventory of your hearts desires. List them as physical goals, mental (creative) goals and spiritual goals. Then, list activities to achieve your goals. To accomplish physical goals, you might list: do yoga or follow a plant-based diet. To accomplish mental peace: you might list, start or continue a hobby that makes you happy. To accomplish spiritual goals: you might help others, be kind and understanding and be a good listener. Who knows, even a smile can lift someone's spirit. Focus on your natural talents to guide your actions to fulfill your goals.

Manifestation meditation: Think of what you want to manifest. Imagine it is here now. Accept that it is yours and that you deserve it and say: I accept.

5

The American Picnic Menu

Beverage~

    Mint Juleps…No alcohol, but lots of mint

Main Course Choices~

    Veggie Patties

    Bean Burgers

    Sweet & Spicy Pears (topping for patties/burgers)

    Cakelike Cornbread

Dessert~

    Baked peaches with granola filling

The American Picnic

BEVERAGE

<u>MINT JULEPS, No alcohol, but lots of mint</u>

Ingredients:

¼ cup fresh mint leaves

½ cup lime juice

½ cup orange juice

4 cups filtered water (not tap water)*

2 tablespoons 100% maple syrup

Method:

Process mint, lime juice and orange juice in a food processor. Strain into a large pitcher (6 cup capacity). Add 4 cups of filtered water and maple syrup and stir to combine. Fill a tall glass with crushed ice and fill glass with mint julip mixture. Add a sprig of mint to garnish.

*Add seltzer water to make this a fizzy drink. Reduce filtered water to 2 cups and add 2 cups of seltzer water.

MAIN COURSE CHOICES

<u>**VEGGIE PATTIES**</u>

Ingredients:

8 ounces diced cooked mushrooms*

1 cup cooked minced onions or 1 teaspoon onion powder

½ teaspoon granulated garlic

1 cup cooked lentils****

1 cup cooked brown rice****

2 tablespoons catsup or tomato sauce

1 tablespoon nutritional yeast**

1 tablespoon dried Italian seasoning

1/8 teaspoon, each salt and black pepper

¼ cup flour

½ cup celery spread or sun-dried tomato dip***

*Acceptable to substitute with 1 cup mashed potatoes

**Substitute ¼ cup plant-based shredded cheese

***Substitute ¼ cup BBQ sauce, pesto or flavor of choice (see Chapter 2 dressings and spreads)

****The brown rice and lentils can be cooked together. In a large sauce pan (8 cup capacity), bring to a boil 4 cups of water. Add 1 cup rice and 1 cup lentils and bring back to a boil. Cover and reduce heat to low and simmer (covered) 45 minutes. This will make more than the 2 cups you need for this recipe, but it freezes well.

Method:
Mix above ingredients in a medium mixing bowl until well combined. Shape into 6 patties. Shallow fry in an olive oil sprayed frying pan 7 to 10 minutes on each side over medium heat or bake on non-stick parchment paper at 350 degrees F for 20 minutes.

To Serve:
Serve on a bun or bread of choice. Add a lettuce leaf, a slice of tomato and condiments of choice: mustard or sweet and spicy pears (see recipe, this Chapter). See Chapter 2 for dressings and spreads ideas.

Health benefits of Lentils: One of the foods eaten by "the long-lived people in the blue zones" is *Lentils.* It is an economical source of low-fat protein; a good source of iron; and an excellent source of fiber, magnesium and folic acid. Protects the heart and bones. It is rich in complex carbohydrates, a nutrient that increases metabolism and helps the body burn fat. It has 16 grams of fiber per cup and 115 calories in ½ cup. Helps with digestion and weight loss.

www.livestrong.com

<u>BEAN BURGERS</u>

Ingredients:

One 15 ounce can of rinsed and drained beans (any beans you like)

1 flax egg (1 tablespoon flaxseed meal dissolved in 3 tablespoons of warm water. Let sit 30 minutes. Stir with a fork until frothy)

1 tablespoon snipped chives

1 clove of minced garlic

1/8 teaspoon, each salt and black pepper

1 tablespoon, each dried parsley & Italian seasoning

¼ cup crushed tortilla chips or flaxseed meal*

Method:

Mix above ingredients in a food processor or mash with a potato masher until well combined; *add 2 tablespoons flour if needed to bind. Chill mixture 30 minutes. Drop a large spoonful of the mixture into a hot skillet sprayed with olive oil. Slightly flatten each burger. Shallow fry on medium heat, 7 minutes per side. Serve topped with sweet and spicy pears.

Health benefits of Beans: A nutrient dense protein food source that controls appetite. Prevents fatty liver. Stabilizes blood sugar levels. Protects against heart attack, stroke and cancer. May lower cholesterol. Good source of fiber.

Medical News Today.com

SWEET AND SPICY PEARS

Ingredients:

1 red pear, sliced thin and cut to a medium dice*

½ cup orange juice

12 ounce package, frozen bell peppers & onions

1 teaspoon olive oil

¼ teaspoon each salt and black pepper

1 tablespoon grainy mustard

1 tablespoon balsamic vinegar

8 drops liquid stevia or 1 teaspoon maple syrup

Method:

In a small saucepan, cover and cook pears and orange juice on medium heat to a boil. Reduce heat to low and simmer 30 minutes. In a medium sized skillet, over medium heat, sauté the frozen bell peppers and onion blend in 1 teaspoon olive oil (or water) until translucent and soft. In a small bowl combine salt, pepper, mustard, vinegar and stevia or maple syrup; stir to make a sauce. In a medium bowl combine cooked pears, bell peppers, onions and sauce. Gently mix to combine. Store in refrigerator 3 days or freeze up to 1 month. A great topping for vege patties or bean burgers.

*Acceptable if pears are not quite ripe.

CAKE-LIKE CORNBREAD

Dry Ingredients:

¾ cup cornmeal (not masa)

1¼ cup flour (gluten free is acceptable)*

2 teaspoons baking powder

1 teaspoon baking soda

Wet Ingredients:

3 flax eggs (see recipe index)

2/3 cup organic plant-based milk

6 ounce carton vanilla almond yogurt

10 drops of liquid stevia **

1/8 cup club soda

Method: Pre-heat oven to 400 degrees F.

Sift dry ingredients into a medium mixing bowl. In a separate medium mixing bowl, combine wet ingredients, stir well. Add wet ingredients to dry ingredients. Stir to combine. Pour batter into a 10 inch X 10 inch baking dish, sprayed with olive oil or Baker's Joy. Bake at 400 degrees F for 21 minutes. Leave in oven 7 minutes with the heat off. It is done when a toothpick inserted in the middle comes out clean. *See Chapter 9.

**or 1 tablespoon 100% maple syrup

DESSERT

<u>BAKED PEACHES WITH GRANOLA FILLING</u>

Ingredients:

1 peach or pear, washed, cut in half, pitted/cored

2 tablespoons granola: homemade recipe follows

2 tablespoons 100% maple syrup

1 tablespoon orange zest

Method: Pre-heat oven to 350 degrees F

Using a grapefruit spoon, hollow out a small divot in the peach or pear half. Fill each half with 1 tablespoon granola. Place peach or pear half on a non- stick parchment paper lined baking sheet or casserole dish sprayed with olive oil. Drizzle 1 tablespoon maple syrup over one filled peach or pear half. Drizzle remaining maple syrup over the other filled peach or pear half. Bake at 350 degrees F for 30 minutes. Garnish with orange zest. Yields two servings.

Health benefits of oranges and orange zest: A food and a medicine. Boosts bone health; reduces inflammation (anti-arthritic); improves good cholesterol; dissolves kidney stones; have anti-cancer properties and boosts weight loss. Orange scent reduces anxiety and improves mood.

Greenmedinfo.com.

HOMEMADE GRANOLA

Ingredients:

1 tablespoon tahini (sesame seed paste) or almond butter

2 tablespoons 100% maple syrup or date syrup*

½ teaspoon vanilla extract

1/8 teaspoon salt

1 tablespoon water

1 teaspoon cinnamon

1 teaspoon ground ginger

1 cup organic rolled oats

Method: Pre-heat oven to 300 degrees F

In a large mixing bowl add above ingredients and stir to mix well. Spread onto a non-stick parchment paper lined baking sheet. Bake at 300 degrees F for 35 minutes. Stir midway through baking. Store in refrigerator three days or freeze up to one month.

*See recipe index

Research into Alzheimer's Disease

The research I have studied about Alzheimer's disease points to reducing the risk of getting Alzheimer's. Todate, there is no cure and no effective treatment.

Dr. Michael Greger, says in his book _How Not to Die,_ Alzheimer's is incurable, but we can reduce the risk via diet and lifestyle changes. Dr. Greger states, that vegetables, legumes (beans, peas, lentils), fruit and whole grains should replace meats and dairy products. He states the same things that cause hardening of the arteries and heart damage also cause Alzheimer's. High LDL cholesterol (due to trans-fats and saturated fats) causes hardening of the arteries. Dr. Greger advises us to eat a plant-based diet to reduce the risk of Alzheimer's. To protect brain cells, add berries, dark leafy greens, grapes, cranberries, deep red and purple fruit and vegetables to our diet. Engage in aerobic exercise. If you have any medical issues, it is advised you check with your doctor about any change in your diet.

Most of the research on Alzheimer's focuses on optimal nutrition. A plant- based diet of colorful, non-starchy, low glycemic fruit and vegetables, including pre-biotics (dandelion greens, plant-based yogurt, jicama, leeks, fermented vegetables), pro-biotics (plant based yogurt, cooked cabbage, low-salt pickles), natural oils (one teaspoon per day), avocados, whole grains, dark chocolate (one ounce per day), nuts and seeds (one tablespoon per day), legumes (beans, peas, lentils) and Vitamin D and B-12 supplements. No meat, No dairy products, No fried foods, No butter, No margarine, No alcohol, No sugar.

Ninety percent of Alzheimer's is caused by diet and lifestyle. The following _super foods_ protect brain cells: pumpkin seeds, nuts, berries, flaxseeds, turmeric, leafy greens, tea, legumes, red grapes, broccoli, pomegranates and lemon balm.

According to Dr. Oz and Dr. Amen, red, yellow and orange fruit and vegetables reduce the risk of Alzheimer's. They recommend adding a little olive oil while cooking these vegetables to help the body convert the carotenoids to vitamin A. They advise that herbs, such as, parsley, sage, rosemary and thyme strengthen connections within the brain. Dr. Amen says that what we eat is either medicine or poison. Heart health is brain health and there is no suffering in getting well. Dr. Amen specifically advises to avoid aluminum cookware and food and beverages in aluminum cans. He recommends we: reduce stress; learn new things; avoid caffeine; socialize; get physical and mental exercise; eat more fiber; and control obesity and diabetes.

Doctors researching Alzheimer's disease include: Dr. Amen, Dr. Oz, Dr. M. Greger, Dr. Nandi, Dr. Arlene Taylor, R. Tanzi, PhD., Dr. Chopra, Dr. Hyman and Dr. Bredesen and they all focus on the following to reduce the risk of getting Alzheimer's disease.

Stress can shrink the brain. Therefore we need to de-stress and not overextend our commitments. Let minor irritations go.

- Follow a plant-based diet.

- Socialize with friends and family.

- Don't make mountains out of mole hills.

- Find ways to relax: gardening, walking or sitting in a beautiful garden.

- Engage in hobbies that make you happy: art, yoga, music, reading, cooking

- Laugh, exercise, and get plenty of sleep.

- Pray, turn things over to God.

- Visit a spa.

- Stay hydrated. Drink 8 glasses of water per day. Avoid sugary drinks.

- Be optimistic (negative self-talk suppresses the immune system).

- Be around happy people.

- Be aware that alcohol, smoking and obesity can cause dementia.

- Develop emotional maturity (are you happy with your life).

- Give back to the planet and to people, making them better for you being here. Be grateful. Gratitude = Health.

- "Diet profoundly influences nerve health and brain function." Dr. Perlmutter

Today's thoughts create your body tomorrow.

Thoughts in the past created your body today.

Professor R. Tanzi and Dr. Chopra

6

The Italian Party Menu

Beverage~

    Fruit fizz sodas

Main Course Choices~

    Watercress artichoke dip

    Caprese toast cups

    Baked pasta

    Baked zucchini flowers

    Cauliflower pizza

    Roasted tomato pesto

Dessert~

    Lemon-Blueberry Tiramisu

The Italian Party

BEVERAGE

<u>FRUIT FIZZ SODAS</u>

Ingredients:

1 cup fresh fruit,*washed, pitted, hulled and cut to a medium dice

1/8 cup orange juice

1 tablespoon date syrup** or 100% maple syrup

Sparkling apple-cranberry 100% juice***

Fruit slices and mint sprigs for garnish

Method:
Process fruit, orange juice and sweetener in a high powered blender or food processor to a smooth puree (strain if peel does not puree). Keep in refrigerator up to 2 days. Yields approximately 1 cup of fruit puree.

*If using blueberries, add 1 teaspoon lemon juice and ½ cup cranberry juice or orange juice before processing the fruit.

To Serve:
In a tall glass, combine ¼ cup fruit puree with ¾ cup sparkling apple-cranberry 100% juice**. Stir and add ice cubes. Garnish with a slice of fruit and a sprig of mint as a stir stick. Yields 4 servings. Offer guests sweeteners of choice to add depending on sweetness of the fruit puree. *Date syrup, see recipe index.

***Acceptable to use sparkling spring water; any flavor that compliments the fruit. For example, pineapple-mango sparkling spring water with mango fruit puree. Try peach flavored sparkling spring water with peaches. There are also several flavors of sparkling apple 100% juice to compliment fruit.

Tart cherry juice contains melatonin and tryptophan for better sleep.

Pomegranate juice helps prevent bone loss, improves mood, increases oxygen flow for better heart health, lowers blood pressure and prevents blood clots.

Greenmedinfo.com

Passion flower tea reduces anxiety.

Use blueberries to sweeten cookies, cakes, and fruit drinks

MAIN COURSE CHOICES

WATERCRESS ARTICHOKE DIP

Ingredients:

½ a bunch of watercress (a handful) blanched

¼ cup plant-based plain unsweetened yogurt or 2 tablespoons tofu mayonnaise or 2 tablespoons tofu sour cream (see recipe index for both recipes)

¼ cup plant-based shredded cheddar cheese

¼ cup plant-based cream cheese

1 teaspoon jarred creamy horseradish

8 artichoke hearts *

Optional stir-ins: 1 tablespoon snipped chives; 1 teaspoon lemon zest; 2 teaspoons lemon juice; 1/8 teaspoon salt and black pepper; ½ teaspoon granulated garlic; 2 stalks celery (minced)

Method:
Process above ingredients in a food processor, until smooth. Yields 1 cup of dip for raw vegetables.

*Jarred, grilled marinated artichokes are mild. Artichokes are high in fiber and contain antioxidants, quercetin and anthocyanins for heart health.

According to Dr. Oz, watercress is the new kale.

CAPRESE TOAST CUPS

Ingredients:

4 slices of bread (any bread you like)

½ cup herbed plant-based cream cheese*

½ cup sun-dried tomato tofu dip**

16 fresh basil leaves or 1 tablespoon dried basil

Method: Pre-heat oven to 350 degrees F

Roll each slice of bread, with a rolling pin to ¼ inch thin. Cut each thin bread slice into fourths. Spray a mini muffin tin with olive oil spray. Fit one thin bread square into each muffin tin space. Spray bread with olive oil spray. Fill each bread square with 1 teaspoon herbed plant-based cream cheese. Bake at 350 degrees F for 15 minutes. Remove from oven. Top each bread square with 1 teaspoon sun-dried tomato dip. Garnish with a basil leaf or sprinkle with dried basil or dollop with ¼ teaspoon of basil pesto.***

*Stir in 1 teaspoon each granulated garlic and Italian seasoning to 4 ounces plant-based cream cheese.

**See Chapter 2 and recipe index. It is acceptable to use sun-dried tomato chutney. See recipe index

***It is acceptable to use jarred or see recipe index for no oil, no cheese, no nuts pesto or recipe for pesto butter

Basil: Limits stress, helps depression, improves mood.

<u>BAKED PASTA</u>

Ingredients:

4 to 6 ounces uncooked pasta*

24 ounces pasta sauce**

2 tablespoons dried oregano

1 teaspoon granulated garlic

1 to 2 cups of any small diced vegetable***

1 tablespoon olive oil

8 plum tomatoes, sliced or 2 zucchini cut into coins

Method: Pre-heat oven to 350 degrees F

In a large bowl, combine above ingredients, except plum tomatoes or zucchini. Stir to combine well. Spray a 9 inch X 13 inch baking dish with olive oil. Pour in pasta vegetable mixture. Top with sliced tomatoes or zucchini coins. Spray with olive oil. Bake at 350 degrees F for 1 hour. This can be served hot or at room temperature. Keep in refrigerator up to 3 days. Re-heat in microwave 1 minute or in oven 10 minutes.

*Rotini or rigatoni pasta works best in this recipe.

**Acceptable to mix canned diced tomatoes,15 ounce, with 9 ounces vegetable broth in lieu of pasta sauce.

***lightly steamed green beans, zucchini, carrots, onions, mushrooms or leftover veges work well.

BAKED ZUCCHINI FLOWERS

Ingredients:

8 zucchini flowers (no zucchini attached)*

1 cup plant-based ricotta cheese**

¼ cup plant-based shredded mozzarella cheese, plus ¼ cup for sprinkling before baking

1 teaspoon each dried basil & Italian seasoning

Method: Pre-heat oven to 350 degrees F

In a small mixing bowl combine seasonings, ricotta and mozzarella cheeses. Stir well. *Remove stamen from flowers. Spoon or pipe 1 tablespoon of cheese filling into zucchini flower. Spray a 10 inch by 10 inch casserole baking dish with olive oil.*** Arrange filled flowers in the dish. Spray flowers with olive oil. Sprinkle flowers with mozzarella cheese. Bake at 350 degrees F for 10 minutes. Serve hot. Makes 4 servings.

Special notes: Flowers may be plated on top of a dollop of pesto sauce or pasta sauce or without sauce. Homemade ricotta cheese (plant-based).** (See recipe index and Chapter 2.) ***Olive oil spray: Fill a spray bottle with ¼ cup olive oil and ¼ cup of water. Spray oil mixture onto food/pans instead of drizzling olive oil onto food/pans.

Basil: An anti-inflammatory for heart health. Potent antioxidant. Aids digestion.

Simplyhealth.io.com

CAULIFLOWER PIZZA

Ingredients:

One 12 ounce package frozen riced cauliflower

½ cup plant-based shredded mozzarella cheese

2 flax eggs (see recipe index)

1/8 teaspoon each salt and black pepper

½ teaspoon Italian seasoning

1/3 cup oat flour or rice flour

Method: Preheat oven to 350 degrees F

Empty thawed package of cauliflower into a medium mixing bowl and microwave (high setting) 4 minutes. Spread cauliflower on non-stick parchment paper lined baking sheet. Spray with olive oil. Bake at 350 degrees F for 15 minutes to dry out the cauliflower. Cool in refrigerator. In a medium mixing bowl, combine above crust ingredients and add cooled cauliflower, mix well. Dollop six rounds of batter onto a non-stick parchment paper lined baking sheet. Flatten to a 4 inch round. Bake at 350 degrees F for 15 minutes. Flip each round and bake 15 more minutes. Cooked crusts can be frozen. To make pizza: top crusts with pasta sauce or roasted tomato pesto (recipe follows), vegetables of choice, a sprinkle of plant-based shredded cheese and bake at 350 degrees F, for 10 minutes until cheese melts.

ROASTED TOMATO PESTO

Ingredients:

1 cup cherry tomatoes, washed and cut in half

1 tablespoon each dried parsley, dried basil, dried Italian seasoning

1 teaspoon granulated garlic

1/8 teaspoon each salt and black pepper

2 tablespoons olive oil

Method: Pre-heat oven to 350 degrees F

Place tomatoes on a non-stick parchment paper lined baking sheet. Drizzle or spray with olive oil. Bake at 350 degrees F for 40 minutes. Tomatoes will be cooked, but not sun-dried. Cool to room temperature.

In a medium mixing bowl mash tomatoes with a potato masher. Add parsley, basil, Italian seasoning, garlic, salt and pepper. Add olive oil and mash again to a chunky sauce. This makes a great topping for pizza crust. It satisfies a craving for pizza flavor. It also makes a great topping for pasta or baked potatoes.

Health benefits of tomatoes: Tomatoes have antioxidant properties. They contain Lycopene, which reduces risk of heart disease and cancer. Tomatoes are a night shade fruit. Good source of Vitamin C and fiber. They decrease inflammation.

Healthline.com

DESSERT

LEMON ~BLUEBERRY TIRAMISU

Ingredients:

1 citrus cake, cut into cubes (see recipe index)

1 cup brewed strong black tea

1½ cups blueberry jam (or any jam you like)**

2 cups blueberries

Filling Ingredients:

8 ounces (1 cup) silken firm tofu, drained

1 tablespoon olive oil

2 ounces plant-based cream cheese

3 tablespoons date syrup* or 100% maple syrup

3 ounces plant-based vanilla almond yogurt

¼ cup almond milk

1 teaspoon vanilla extract

Method:
Process filling ingredients in a food processor, until smooth.

*See recipe index or recipe below

Method for each layer: Two layers
In a 9 inch X 9 inch casserole dish, layer cake cubes in a single layer. Drizzle half the cooled brewed black tea over cake cubes. Spread half the jam over the cake cubes. Spoon half the filling over the jam and smooth to cover the cake to fit the dish.

Sprinkle half the blueberries over the filling. Repeat the above layer, ending with blueberries on top. Keep refrigerated Yields 8 servings.

****No-cook blueberry jam:**

  1 pound blueberries, fresh or frozen.

  2 tablespoons lemon juice

  2 tablespoons ground chia seeds

  3 tablespoons date syrup ***

Method:
Combine above ingredients in a medium mixing bowl. Mash with a potato masher to a smooth consistency. Cover and chill 1 hour. Keep in refrigerator up to 3 days.

*****Lemon date syrup**: 8 pitted dates plumped in 1 cup boiling water. Cool. Cut up 1 lemon, including rind. Process dates, water and lemon in a blender or food processor to a smooth puree. Keep in refrigerator up to 3 days or freeze one month.

Foods that Fight Inflammation

We can be healthy as we age. Learn how to use food as medicine. Make health your first priority. Quality of life improves on a plant-based diet: creating less depression, more energy, weight loss, potential reversal of disease, less anxiety, less neuropathy. Inflammation is defined as: a red, swollen, hot, painful, inflamed part of the body due to injury or infection. Inflammation is the body's immune response to injury, viruses and bacteria. It is the body's attempt to heal itself after an injury and defend itself against viruses, bacteria and damaged tissue.

Nutritionists advise that the following foods fight inflammation:

- Omega 3 fatty acids, such as: flaxseed meal, avocados, chia seeds, nuts, seeds and borage.
- Cruciferous vegetables, such as: broccoli and kale.
- Green leafy vegetables.
- Onions.
- Olive oil. Berries.
- Whole grains, such as: brown rice, quinoa, organic rolled oats.
- Cocoa powder.
- Mushrooms.
- Tomatoes.
- Fruit.
- Legumes such as: beans, peas and lentils.
- Tea.
- Stevia and date syrup.
- Herbs and spices such as: ginger, garlic, cloves, rosemary, turmeric, oregano, nutmeg.

The foods listed above build the immune system and stop inflammation.

Foods that cause inflammation include: acidic foods: red meat, processed meats, butter, lard, shortening, soda, beverages sweetened with sugar, fried foods, dairy products, cheese, ice cream, refined carbohydrates, white bread and pastries. Pollen, chemicals and microbes can also cause an immune response.

It's nice to have a list of foods that fight inflammation. With planning and recipes, you can create appetizing, nutritionally dense, anti-inflammatory dishes that you and your family enjoy. You can educate yourself about how to adapt an *inflammatory* recipe into an *anti-inflammatory* recipe by knowing healthy food substitutes. My recipes and many plant-based cookbooks can teach you how to prepare food for health, even ice cream (see my recipe index).

7

The Mexican Fiesta Menu

Beverage~

Blueberry Mojitos (no alcohol, but lots of mint)

Main Course~

Tin foil tamales

Green chili enchiladas, adapted from my sister Mary's recipe

Grandma's homemade mild salsa

Dessert~

Strawberry cake (In honor of grandma)

Sweet potato ice cream (vanilla)

The Mexican Fiesta

BEVERAGE

<u>BLUEBERRY MOJITOS~(mint, no alcohol)</u>

Ingredients

- 1 cup blueberry- pomegranate juice (Knudsen's)
- 1 cup mint overnight tea*
- 1 cup mint water**
- ¼ cup lime juice
- ½ cup sparkling lime mineral water
- 2 tablespoons 100% maple syrup or date syrup**
- 1 cup filtered water (not tap water)

Method:
*In a 6 cup capacity pitcher (lidded) place 3 mint tea bags in 4 cups filtered water. Refrigerate overnight. Discard tea bags. This makes crystal clear overnight mint tea. **Mint water: combine 20 mint leaves in a blender with 3 cups of overnight mint tea. Blend well and strain out the mint leaves (or not). In a 6 cup capacity pitcher combine blueberry juice, 1 cup mint tea, 1cup mint water, lime juice, mineral water, sweetener and 1 cup filtered water. Stir well.

To serve:

Serve mojito mixture in a tall glass over ice. Garnish with a sprig of mint. Yields 4 servings. You may freeze the extra 2 cups of mint tea.

Health benefits of mint: Mint has the highest antioxidant levels of any food. Relieves seasonal allergy symptoms. It is a decongestant. Aids digestion and flatulence. Is a natural antimicrobial and breath freshener. It can increase motivation and uplift mood. It can increase alertness. Helps with memory. Lowers appetite and helps with overeating. Boosts vitality. Helps with migraines.

Medical News today.com

Health benefits of blueberries: Blueberries have the highest amount of antioxidants of any fruit. They are a good source of fiber, Vitamin C, potassium, folate, and Vitamin B-6. They have a high anthocyanin content. Can protect against cancer and heart disease. They have calcium and magnesium which help maintain bone strength. They may help improve short-term memory. They may lower blood pressure, improve blood sugar and insulin levels. Slows cognitive decline.

WebMD.com

Health benefits of citrus: A concentrated source of Vitamin C. Helps support heart health. Reduces risk of asthma. Promotes healthy skin. Increases energy. Boosts the immune system (has antibacterial and antifungal properties). Helps build and maintain collagen (less wrinkles). Lowers risk of stroke.

Medical news today.com.

MAIN COURSE

<u>TIN FOIL TAMALES</u>

Dough, dry ingredients:

½ cup masa (Maseca, instant corn masa flour)

1/8 cup cornmeal

½ teaspoon baking powder

Dough, wet ingredients:

2 tablespoons olive oil

¾ cup mild canned green enchilada sauce (this can be spicy. Acceptable to mix ¼ cup green enchilada sauce with ½ cup water.)

Method:
Sift dry ingredients into a medium mixing bowl. Stir in wet ingredients. Mix to a soft paste. Let rest 5 minutes.

Filling ingredients:

¼ cup cooked beans (canned are acceptable) (any beans you like)

¼ cup cooked brown rice

2 tablespoons cooked diced onions

¼ cup salsa (any salsa you like)

¼ cup chopped green chilies (use canned)

½ cup plant-based shredded cheddar cheese

Method:

Mix above filling ingredients in a small mixing bowl.

To assemble:

Cut 6 tin foil bases, 6 inches wide X 12 inches long. Cut 6 non-stick parchment paper bases, 6 inches wide X 12 inches long. Lay each parchment paper base on top of each tin foil base. Spoon a smear of masa dough 3 inches wide X 4 inches long onto each parchment paper base. Spoon filling 1 inch wide down the center of each dough smear. Roll masa dough over the filling (use parchment paper to help roll the dough over the filling) to completely enclose the filling inside the masa dough. Fold parchment paper over dough and fold ends of parchment paper, like a flap at each end to create a packet. Fold the tin foil over the parchment paper, and fold ends of tin foil like a flap at each end to create a packet. Place each packet standing up in a lidded steamer basket. Steam 30 minutes, with lid on. Let rest 15 minutes to set-up. Serve topped with salsa. Yields 6 tamales.

Health benefits of green chilies: Rich in fiber (helps digestion). Has Vitamin C (immune system) which can combat colds and sinus infections. The heat from the chilies is an effective pain reliever. Can reduce atherosclerosis, cholesterol and triglycerides. Zero calories.

food.ndtv.com

GREEN CHILI ENCHILADAS ADAPTED FROM MY SISTER MARY'S RECIPE

Ingredients for the filling:

2 cups cooked brown rice

½ cup cooked lentils

1 cup cooked diced celery

¼ cup cooked onions or 1 teaspoon onion powder

Ingredients for the sauce:

2 cups mild green enchilada sauce (canned)

½ cup bottled tomatillo salsa

2½ cups of water

Ingredients for topping and layering:

8 ounce package, plant-based shredded cheese

A package of corn tortillas

Method: Pre-heat oven to 350 degrees F

In a large lidded saucepan, add 1 cup rice, ½ cup lentils, 1 cup celery and ¼ cup chopped onions to 3 cups boiling water. Stir to combine. Reduce heat to low and simmer, lidded, 45 minutes. Yields 6 cups rice/lentil mixture. Wrap 12 corn tortillas in a paper towel and microwave (on high) 1 minute to soften. In a medium mixing bowl, combine sauce ingredients. Stir. Spray a deep casserole baking dish (8 inch X 8 inch X 3 inches deep) with olive oil. Spoon 1/3 cup sauce on bottom of baking dish. Dip 2 tortillas in sauce and place in a single layer on the bottom of baking dish (acceptable to tear tortillas into fourths to fit the baking dish). Top tortillas with 2 cups rice, lentil, celery and onion mixture. Spoon 1/3 cup sauce over rice mixture. Sprinkle 1/3 cup plant-based shredded cheese over rice mixture. Continue with 2 more layers: sauced tortillas, rice mixture, enchilada sauce, cheese, ending with rice mixture, sauce &cheese on top. Bake, uncovered, at 350 degrees F for 40 minutes. Yields 8 servings.

Mole sauce can be substituted for green chili sauce:
1 tablespoon onion powder
2 teaspoons granulated garlic
2 teaspoons lime juice
2 teaspoons chili powder (any type you like)
½ teaspoon each dried cumin, cinnamon, oregano, coriander
2 tablespoons flour or Bisquick baking mix
2 cups vegetable stock
1 tablespoon almond butter
2 tablespoons catsup
2 tablespoons cocoa powder
1 tablespoon jarred Dona Maria mole sauce (purchase at grocery store) dissolved in ¼ cup hot water

Method: Combine above ingredients in a medium saucepan and cook on low heat 20 minutes. Stir frequently. If sauce is too thick add 1 cup water or vegetable stock. This is a mild quick mole that works well for dipping the corn tortillas and adding sauce to the enchiladas. This sauce can be made spicier by adding 1 more tablespoon of Dona Maria jarred mole sauce dissolved in ¼ cup hot water.

GRANDMA'S HOMEMADE MILD SALSA

Ingredients:

½ of a 15 ounce can petite diced tomatoes + juice

½ of a 4 ounce can of diced mild green chilies

1 scallion, chopped or 6 chives, snipped

1/8 teaspoon each salt and black pepper

1 teaspoon balsamic vinegar

1 teaspoon olive oil

4 drops, liquid stevia or ½ teaspoon maple syrup

Method:
Combine above ingredients in a small mixing bowl. Keep refrigerated up to 3 days. Yields, about 1 cup.

DESSERTS

STRAWBERRY CAKE

Dry Ingredients:

1 cup flour*

1 teaspoon baking soda

½ teaspoon cardamom**(optional)

1 teaspoon cinnamon

1/8 teaspoon salt (optional)

1 packet of powered stevia

Wet Ingredients:

¼ cup beet juice from a 15 ounce can of shoestring red beets

¼ cup date syrup (see recipe index)

1 teaspoon strawberry or vanilla extract

1 flax egg (see recipe index)

¼ cup plant-based vanilla almond yogurt

1 tablespoon olive oil

*See Chapter 10, baking without wheat flour, for various no-wheat flour combinations.

**Cardamom can give a soapy taste. Acceptable to omit.

Stir-ins:

1 tablespoon orange zest

1 cup chopped canned shoestring red beets

½ cup pureed strawberries*

½ cup fresh or frozen blueberries

Method: Pre-heat oven to 375 degrees F
Sift dry ingredients into a medium mixing bowl. Combine wet ingredients in a small mixing bowl. Add wet ingredients to dry ingredients and mix well. Stir in beets, strawberry puree*, orange zest and blueberries. Mix well. Pour batter into a 9 inch X 9 inch baking dish sprayed with olive oil. Bake at 375 degrees F for 30 minutes. Cool completely before cutting. Frost with gold sweet potato frosting and serve with gold sweet potato ice cream.

*In a food processor, puree 1 pound fresh or 1 bag frozen, thawed strawberries. Keep any leftover puree in the freezer for one month.

Health benefits of strawberries: Contains Vitamin C, manganese, folate, potassium and antioxidants for heart health and blood sugar control. Lowers blood pressure; maintains eye health; helps arthritis symptoms; increases metabolism. *Healthline.com*

This cake is an homage to my grandmother, who ate strawberries every day and lived to age 97.

SWEET POTATO ICE CREAM (VANILLA)

Ingredients:

1 large baked gold sweet potato (skin removed)*

1½ cups plant-based milk**

1 teaspoon vanilla extract or vanilla bean seeds

¼ cup plant-based vanilla yogurt

2 tablespoons 100% maple syrup***

Method:
Combine above ingredients in a food processor and process until very smooth. Place in the freezer to freeze. Yields 2 cups soft serve ice cream. If you have an ice cream machine place processed ingredients in the machine and process for 20 minutes. Should be the consistency of ice cream. Keep in freezer. Thaw 30 minutes to serve as ice cream.

*Gold or Hannah sweet potatoes have tan skin and cream color flesh. Wrap in foil, place on a baking sheet. Bake at 400 degrees F for 1 hour. Test with a cake tester. Cool. Remove skin.

**Unsweetened organic vanilla almond milk is thicker than most plant-based milk and works well in this recipe.

***10 drops of liquid stevia may be substituted for maple syrup. Gold sweet potatoes are naturally sweet.

Special note: 1 cup blueberries or strawberries or 1 banana or ¼ cup cocoa powder may be added to this recipe to change the flavor.

This is a true story about a healing miracle and forgiveness. I have been an acupressure therapist for 30 years. People come to me for treatments for pain relief.

A man in his 60's was brought to me by his wife because he was experiencing pain in his right shoulder. He suffered with this pain all his life and sought a diagnosis and treatment from many doctors. The doctors told him there was nothing wrong and there was no treatment, but still the pain persisted.

I started the acupressure treatment and soon a woman's spirit appeared to me. I described her to the man and asked if he knew her. He said no, he had never seen her and did not know her. I continued the treatment and the woman's spirit appeared a second time. Again the man said he had never met her and didn't know her. The third time the woman's spirit appeared I was working on the man's shoulder. Finally the man said, "oh yes, I know her, she is my grandmother, my father's mother." I said, she wants you to forgive her. The man recalled an incident when he was 9 or 10 years old. He had an argument with his father. The boy was so upset, he ran away from home. He was gone 2 or 3 days. When he returned home, his grandmother opened the front door and instead of welcoming him home, she slapped him in the face very hard and said "your father has been worried sick about you, don't you ever run away again."

I asked him if he would be willing to say the forgiveness prayer for her. He agreed. He and I said the forgiveness prayer for her. Suddenly, while I was still holding his ailing shoulder and while saying the forgiveness prayer, there was a loud popping sound, like air whooshing out of his shoulder and the man said: "all the pain is gone."

His wife, who was sitting across the room, started saying "it's a miracle, it's a miracle." According to his wife, the pain never returned.

Now, I offer the forgiveness prayer to you. I received this prayer during a live channeling session where June Burke channeled the teaching of Archangel *Julian*, granting us his knowledge. Here is Archangel *Julian's* forgiveness prayer (paraphrased):

Forgiveness Prayer

Visualize and name the person you are forgiving

<u>Name:</u> *I forgive you for anything bad I think you ever did to me*

and

I ask that you forgive me for anything bad you think I ever did to you.

I bless you, I forgive you, I wish you well.

If you are never going to see or talk to the person again, add this part of the prayer:

I release you to the past, you cannot come forward with me, you must stay in the past.

June Burke is in Heaven. *Julian,* the Archangel does not channel through anyone anymore.

Forgiveness is a process. You may have to say the forgiveness prayer 100 times for the same person. Say it every time you think of the person you need to forgive. Forgiveness releases our resentments. If you want to talk about what the other person did to you, say the forgiveness prayer instead.

I have discovered we can forgive people, places, issues, everyone and everything that has ever kicked sand in our face.

Forgive for your heart's sake. Letting go of anger has dramatic fast acting health benefits. Anger puts your nervous system on high alert. Forgiving helps us feel calm and in control. Anger creates stress that reduces our immune system. Don't expect an apology. No one can change the past. You can take responsibility for healing yourself. When we wish others well, it replaces bitterness with a positive emotion. Repeat the forgiveness prayer as needed when painful memories replay.

Prevention Magazine.

8

Sweet Treats Choices

Beverages~

  Strawberry basil cooler

  Hot cocoa

Sweet treats choices~

  Pumpkin pie cookies

  Pumpkin cake

  Sweet velvet pumpkin pie

  Cake-like brownies

  Fudge-like brownies

  Carrot cake

Life is uncertain, Eat dessert first. Ernestine Ulmer

Sweet Treats Choices

BEVERAGES

<u>STRAWBERRY BASIL COOLER</u>

Ingredients:

½ pound of strawberries (about 10), rinsed, hulled and quartered

1 tablespoon 100% maple syrup or date syrup

2 large basil leaves

1 teaspoon lime juice, fresh or bottled

¼ cup good quality water

Method:
Process above ingredients in a high powered blender or food processor until strawberries are a smooth puree. Add strawberry puree to a large pitcher (6 cup capacity), add ice cubes and 3 cups of good quality water. Stir. Serve over ice in a tall glass. Garnish with a strawberry. Yields 4 servings.

Health benefits of strawberries: They whiten teeth and protect skin against sunburn.

Prevention magazine

HOT COCOA

Ingredients:

2 cups plant-based milk *

1 tablespoon cocoa powder or cacao powder **

10 drops of liquid stevia ***

Method:

In a medium sized saucepan, heat above ingredients. Stir well. When hot and all the cocoa powder has been dissolved and absorbed, stir again. Ladle into small heat proof cups. Yields 4 servings, about ½ cup each. Refrigerate any leftover hot cocoa to drink as chocolate milk when cold.

*Organic, unsweetened vanilla almond milk works best.

**Cocoa powder is raw cacao that has been roasted at high temperatures (reducing enzyme counts). Cacao powder is cold-pressed, unroasted cacao beans, which keeps living enzymes in the cacao). *Foodmatters.com*

***Acceptable to use 1 tablespoon 100% maple syrup

Health benefits of Cacao: Contains Resveratrol, a potent antioxidant that protects the nervous system and boosts mood. Dairy milk inhibits the absorption of antioxidants from raw cacao.

Foodmatters.com

SWEET TREATS CHOICES

PUMPKIN PIE COOKIES

Dry Ingredients:

¾ cup organic rolled oats

½ teaspoon baking powder (aluminum free)

1/8 teaspoon baking soda

½ teaspoon pumpkin pie spice

Wet Ingredients:

1 flax egg (see recipe index)

½ cup pumpkin puree or sweet potato puree

1 tablespoon date syrup* or applesauce

1 tablespoon olive oil

½ teaspoon vanilla extract

Optional Stir-ins: 1/3 cup mini chocolate chips, or dried cranberries or blueberries (fresh or frozen).

Method: Pre-heat oven to 350 degrees F

In a medium mixing bowl mix dry ingredients. In a small bowl mix wet ingredients. Add wet ingredients to dry ingredients and add optional stir-ins, mix well. On a non-stick parchment paper lined baking sheet, drop dough by tablespoons & slightly flatten. Bake at 350 degrees F for 18 to 20 minutes. Yields 12 to 14 cookies. *See recipe index

Juice combinations to make you look younger:

<u>Apple carrot juice:</u>

1 apple

1 inch ginger root, peeled

1 carrot (medium dice)

1 cup of greens (dandelion, sorrel, lettuce, spinach, or any green vegetable you like).

Process above ingredients in a food processor or blender to juice consistency. Add 2 cups of spring water to thin. Makes 4 servings.

<u>Carrot lemon juice:</u>

1 carrot (medium dice)

Juice of 1 lemon

1 cup of greens (any green vegetable you like)

Process above ingredients in a food processor or blender to juice consistency. Add 2 cups of spring water to thin. Makes 4 servings.

Dandelions help with arthritis pain and Fibromialgia pain.

<u>PUMPKIN CAKE</u>

Dry Ingredients:

1 cup flour

½ teaspoon baking soda

½ teaspoon each cinnamon, cardamom, pumpkin pie spice, salt and vanilla bean seeds

Wet Ingredients:

¼ cup date syrup* or applesauce

¾ cup pumpkin puree or sweet potato puree

1/3 cup plant-based yogurt

1 tablespoon olive oil

2 tablespoons 100% maple syrup

1 flax egg (see recipe index)

Method: Pre-heat oven to 350 degrees F

This is a dense bake and can be used as a cake or a bread. Sift dry ingredients into a medium mixing bowl. Mix wet ingredients in a separate medium mixing bowl. Add wet ingredients to dry ingredients. Spray an 8 inch X 8 inch baking dish with olive oil or Baker's Joy. Pour batter into prepared dish and spread batter to be level in the dish. Bake at 350 degrees F for 30 minutes. Cool and frost with sweet potato frosting. Yields 16 servings. *See recipe index

SWEET VELVET PUMPKIN PIE

Ingredients: Filling is for one pie crust

¾ cup canned pumpkin puree (unsweetened)

4 ounces plant-based cream cheese

¼ cup 100% maple syrup or date syrup*

1 teaspoon pumpkin pie spice

1/8 teaspoon salt (optional)

1 flax egg (see recipe index)

¼ cup plant based milk

¼ cup plant based yogurt (vanilla flavor)

1 teaspoon vanilla extract

Method: Pre-heat oven to 350 degrees F

In a food processor, process above ingredients until it is a silky, smooth puree. Pour filling into an unbaked pie shell (store bought is acceptable). Sprinkle lightly with ground cinnamon. Place pie on a baking sheet. After 15 minutes of baking, cover crust edges with tin foil or a metal crust ring. Bake at 350 degrees F for 55 minutes. (Pie will be a little giggly in the middle, but will set-up in the refrigerator). Chill 24 hours before cutting. Top with mock **Devonshire cream.**

Mock Devonshire cream:

12 ounces silken extra firm tofu, ¼ cup 100% maple syrup and ½ teaspoon vanilla extract. Process in a food processor.

<u>CAKE-LIKE BROWNIES</u>

Dry Ingredients:

1 cup flour

2 tablespoons cacao powder or cocoa powder

1 teaspoon baking powder

1/3 cup plant-based chocolate chips

Wet Ingredients

2 tablespoons date syrup or applesauce

½ cup plant-based milk

1/8 cup prune puree (jarred baby food)

2 tablespoons olive oil

½ cup sweet potato puree or pumpkin puree

1 tablespoon apple juice or cranberry juice

1 teaspoon vanilla extract

Method: Pre-heat oven to 350 degrees F.

Sift dry ingredients into a medium mixing bowl. Stir in chocolate chips. Mix well. In a large mixing bowl, combine wet ingredients. Mix well. Add dry ingredients to wet ingredients. Mix well. Spoon batter into an 8 inch X 8 inch baking dish, sprayed with Baker's Joy. Bake at 350 degrees F for 30 minutes. Chill well before cutting.

FUDGE-LIKE BROWNIES

Dry Ingredients

½ cup flour

2 tablespoons cocoa powder

¼ teaspoon salt (optional)

¼ teaspoon baking soda

½ cup plant based chocolate chips

Wet Ingredients:

1 tablespoon olive oil

3 tablespoons date syrup or applesauce

1 flax egg (see recipe index)

½ cup pumpkin puree

2 teaspoons vanilla extract

Method: Pre-heat oven to 350 degrees F.

Combine wet ingredients in a medium mixing bowl. Stir well to blend. Add sifted dry ingredients, mix well. Spoon batter into an 8 inch X 8 inch baking dish sprayed with Bakers Joy. Bake at 350 degrees F for 25 minutes. Chill and cut with a serrated knife. Top with chocolate **sweet potato frosting**:

Sweet Potato Frosting: Mash 1 cooked, peeled orange sweet potato. Stir in 2 tablespoons cocoa powder. Mix until consistency of frosting. Keep refrigerated.

CARROT CAKE

Dry Ingredients:

1 cup flour

1 teaspoon baking soda

1 teaspoon each cardamom* and cinnamon

¼ teaspoon salt (optional) (see Chapter 9)

Wet Ingredients:

1 tablespoon orange zest

¼ cup cranberry or orange juice

1 tablespoon 100% maple syrup

1 flax egg (see recipe index)**

¼ cup plant-based vanilla yogurt

1 tablespoon olive oil

Stir-ins:

1 cup grated raw carrots

½ cup blueberries or cranberries

*It is mentioned in Dr. Michael Greger's book, _How not to Die,_ that the spice cardamom kills cancer cells.

**Acceptable to mix the flaxseed meal with the cranberry juice so cake does not get soggy.

Method: Pre-heat oven to 375 degrees F.

Sift dry ingredients into a medium mixing bowl. Combine wet ingredients in a small mixing bowl. Bend well. Add wet ingredients to dry ingredients. Stir in carrots & fruit. Blend well. Pour into a 9 inch X 9 inch or 9 inch X 13 inch baking dish sprayed with Bakers Joy. Bake at 375 degrees F for 25 minutes until a toothpick inserted in the middle comes out clean. When cooled and well chilled, cut with a serrated knife. *Adapted from Health.com.* Frost with plant based cream cheese frosting.

Plant-based cream cheese frosting: 2 ounces plant based cream cheese, 2 tablespoons plant-based vanilla yogurt, 2 tablespoons 100% maple syrup and 1 teaspoon lime juice. Process in food processor until smooth. Thinly spread on top of carrot cake.

Embarrassing Moments

This is a true story. I call it meltdown at the museum. My friend Lee (not her real name) and I were at the Regan Library in Simi Valley. We went through the first part of the museum and down a long hallway to an octagon shaped room on our right. The lights in the room were dim and the walls were navy blue with white writing and pictures on them. Lee opened a door and was 3 or 4 paces ahead of me. A museum docent stepped between Lee and me and said to me "you can't go in there". There were a lot of people in the octagon room. I started to feel claustrophobic, like I couldn't get any air. Then, I felt tightness in my chest. The feeling of not being able to breathe got worse. I said to the docent, I have to get out of here, I can't breathe. The docent said "I can't open the door until the film in the next room is finished which won't be for another 30 seconds". I told the docent again, I had to get out of the room as I felt faint, like I was going to pass out. The docent still would not open the door. I looked behind me and there were people shoulder to shoulder at least 10 people deep. Just then, the door opened and Lee pulled me into the next room. She pulled me by the arm through the length of the room to an open hallway with benches along the wall. I sat down to catch my breath. She asked me what was wrong. I told her I couldn't breathe. Lee asked if I knew where we had just been? I said no. Lee said those two rooms were all about the assassination attempt on President Regan and the movie they were showing in the room I was in was all about them wheeling President Regan down the hallway to surgery. I said I was re-living President Regan's pain and not being able to breathe. I told Lee they should post a sign on the door to not enter if you are an empath.

If you have a frightening experience, ask for God's white light of protection.

The following protection prayer (paraphrased) was given to me by one of my mentors, Brett Bravo, a renowned healer and author of several books on healing.

The white light of divine protection surrounds me now, sealing out all negative experiences. Only goodness can enter this wonderful light and I will send only goodness out through it. Thank you heavenly Father for your perfect protection.

9

Probiotics and Prebiotics
Complimentary Proteins
Substitutes for oil and eggs

Probiotics: Provides good bacteria for the intestines, the immune system and for healing leaky gut. It replenishes good bacteria. Antibiotics kill these good bacteria. *WebMD.com*

Probiotic foods include: Plant-based yogurt, marinated vegetables, pickled cucumbers, Miso, Dark Chocolate, Olives, Apple Cider Vinegar, Green Peas and pickles.

Prebiotics: Help digest food for healthy intestines. They are types of dietary fiber that feed the probiotic bacteria. *WebMD.com*

Prebiotic foods include: Onions/leeks, Asparagus, Green Leafy Vegetables, Bananas, Apples, Jicama, Oats. Beans, Berries, Whole grains, Cabbage, Legumes, Cocoa powder, Garlic, Barley, Flaxseeds and Dandelions.

Complementary Proteins

Many people are concerned about not getting enough protein from a plant based diet. However, there are ways to combine plant foods so you get adequate protein in your diet without eating meat and dairy products.

In her 1982 edition of _Diet for a small planet,_ Frances Lappe states: "with a healthy varied diet, concern about protein complementarity is not necessary for most of us......however, complementary protein combinations evolved spontaneously as the basis of virtually all the world's great cuisines."

In 1972, Dr. Edmund S. Nasset, a research physiologist, published an article titled, "The Role of the Digestive System in Protein Metabolism", in which he reported evidence of an "amino acid pool that could make up for any deficiencies in the amino acid patterns of the food we eat."

On Dr. Michael Greger's website, _Nutritionfacts.org.,_ Dr. Greger advises that "all essential amino acids originate from plants and microbes, and all plant proteins contain all the essential amino acids. Our bodies maintain pools of free amino acids that can be used to do all the protein complementing for us. All the essential amino acids are circulating in our blood stream and they know how to combine on their own to make a complete protein. We do not need to be concerned about amino acid imbalance."

However, according to Ayurvedic and Chinese medicine, if you combine the wrong foods, your body will become acidic and unbalanced. Your digestion will suffer.

Therefore, to promote a healthy digestive system, the following are food combinations to consider. They provide all the essential amino acids to make a complete protein.

Foods that combine to become a complete protein:

Any grain combined with any green vegetable.

Rice, breads, cereals, grains, oats, corn + vegetables.

Rice, breads, cereals, grains, oats, corn + Legumes.

Rice, breads, cereals, grains, oats, corn + nuts & seeds

Legumes are peas, lentils, beans.

Note: Quinoa is a complete protein. There are 14 grams of protein in ½ cup.

Edamame, Tofu, and Soybeans are complete proteins. There are 11 grams of protein in 1/3 cup.

Advanced food combining:

Almonds + Soy.

Kidney beans + sesame seeds.

Lima beans + brown rice

Oatmeal + wheat germ.

Dates + leafy greens.

Beets + beans. (See recipe for beet humus)

Grains + beans.

Vitamin G: which means gardening in the sunshine for 5 minutes can lead to well- being and feeling better.

Many of the recipes in this book combine foods for good digestion. See the recipe index for pasta salad with vegetables; Enchiladas (made with rice and lentils); or baked pasta with vegetables.

Top 10 fruit and vegetables to add to your diet:

Kale (blanched or sautéed 5 minutes)

Prunes (Dried Plums)

Raisins

Blueberries

Oranges

Strawberries

Spinach

Brussel Sprouts

Broccoli

Alfalfa Sprouts

Broccoli Sprouts

Substitutes for oil and eggs

Substitutes for oil:

<u>In pesto</u>: In a recipe, to omit *all* the oil, tahini, cheese and nuts, use ½ cup cooked brown rice or cooked quinoa. This will give a creamy texture without any oil product.

<u>In breads and cakes:</u> To omit *all* the oil in a recipe, use a fruit puree, such as: prune puree (see recipe index) or (buy jarred baby food), applesauce or banana puree. I have replaced all the oil in a recipe with equal amounts of applesauce, or banana, or prune puree without baking problems. Example: replace 1/3 cup butter or oil with 1/3 cup fruit puree.*

<u>In scones and cookies (even ice cream):</u> Omit *all* the oil by using almond yogurt, tofu, pureed sweet potato, pumpkin puree, or pureed mashed white potatoes.

<u>In any recipe:</u> Omit *all* the oil by using tahini or almond butter.

Special notes: If the final product is too dense or too dry, add ¼ cup club soda for a lighter texture or you may add 1 teaspoon to 1 tablespoon olive oil and try the recipe again. Using date syrup (a fruit puree, see recipe index) as your sweetener cuts the amount of oil needed.*

<u>Fruit puree recipe</u>: Bring 1 cup pitted dried fruit (apricots, dates, dried plums, peaches, etc.) and I cup water to a boil. Reduce heat to low and simmer 10 minutes. Add ½ teaspoon vanilla extract. Cool and process to a smooth puree in a food processor.

Substitutes for eggs:

<u>To substitute one egg in a recipe:</u>

1 flax egg* (see recipe index). If the recipe calls for other liquids, mix the flaxseed meal with that liquid, so the baked item does not get soggy.

¼ cup applesauce

½ a ripe banana (mashed)

1 teaspoon almond butter + 1/8 cup almond milk

1 tablespoon vinegar +1 teaspoon baking soda, let fizz

¼ cup almond yogurt

¼ cup fruit puree

¼ cup tofu, processed until smooth

Egg Replacer: Ener-G egg replacer found at Health food stores

3 tablespoons aqua faba (canned bean water)

1 tablespoon ground chia seeds dissolved in 3 tablespoons water; let stand 15 minutes

2 tablespoons flour + ½ teaspoon oil

1½ tablespoons plant based sour cream

Flax egg: 1 tablespoon flaxseed meal dissolved in 3 tablespoons of warm water. Let sit 15 to 30 minutes, then stir with a fork until frothy. Add to wet ingredients

*I use the flax egg. It adds a nut-like flavor to the bake.

Plant-based substitutes for:

1 cup Buttermilk: 1 cup plant-based yogurt or almond milk + 1 tablespoon lemon juice

1 cup Yogurt: 1 cup fruit puree

1 cup Heavy cream: 2/3 cup almond milk + 1/3 cup plant-based melted margarine or olive oil.

Omitting salt in a recipe:

Salt is a flavor enhancer. It has a strengthening effect on the gluten protein in the dough. In gluten free baking, salt may be omitted. Without salt, your cake won't taste as sweet and may even taste flat. Cookies without salt may taste too sweet. However, for salt sensitive individuals, I leave the salt out of the recipe and find no difference in taste.

Adding flavor without salt:

For savory recipes, use pesto, carrots, celery, onions, tomatoes, and zucchini.

To sweeten and moisten cakes and cookies, use blueberries, carrots, cranberries, zucchini and diced cooked fruit.

Intuition class

This is a true story. While I was working at my tea garden in Vista, I noticed the tenant left a glass on a serving table. I didn't want the glass to get broken in the garden, so I took it into the laundry room. As soon as I put the glass down on the washing machine, intuition said: "take the glass into the kitchen". I don't normally go into the tenant's kitchen, unless I'm hosting a high tea. But, since no one was home, I took the glass into the kitchen and set it on the drain board. As I reached across the stove, I sensed heat coming from the oven. I opened the oven door and saw that the broiler was on. The broiler pan and drippings were sizzling (maybe from meat cooked for breakfast). I turned off the broiler. Had I not listened to my intuition, I'm sure there would have been a kitchen fire.

The message from this experience is that there is *divine intervention* (we call it intuition) to guide and help us. We should always listen to our intuition even if it will inconvenience us or sound silly to us. It may save us from a dire situation. Your intuition will always tell you the truth about people, places and situations.

10

No Wheat Recipe choices

No wheat cornbread

No wheat bread

Chocolate chip blueberry cookies

Sweet potato scones

Strawberry rice cake treats

Oatmeal Cake-like scones

Chocolate oatmeal cake

Date cake

So soft chocolate chip oat cookies

Matcha green tea cookies

Sugar-free fruit fudge

Special note: Baking with rice flour, oat flour, quinoa flour*
and buckwheat flour (a wheat free seed), replaces wheat flour.
Individuals sensitive to gluten, cannot have wheat flour. Replace
1 cup wheat flour with ½ cup oat flour + ¼ cup quinoa flour +
¼ cup rice flour. This can be a used as rice flour baking mix.
Many doctors say that wheat causes inflammation in the body.
*Grind uncooked quinoa in a coffee grinder to make a flour

<u>NO WHEAT CORNBREAD</u>

Dry Ingredients:

½ cup organic rolled oats

1 cup cornmeal

2 teaspoons baking powder

1 teaspoon onion powder

½ teaspoon salt (optional)

Wet Ingredients:

2 flax eggs (see recipe index)

1 cup plant-based milk

2 tablespoons olive oil

Method: Pre-heat oven to 375 degrees F

Mix dry ingredients in a large mixing bowl. Add wet ingredients. Stir well to combine. Pour batter into a Bundt pan or 9 inch X 9 inch baking dish sprayed with olive oil. Bake at 375 degrees F for 30 minutes, until a toothpick inserted in the middle comes out clean.

<u>NO WHEAT BREAD</u>

Dry Ingredients:

½ cup oat flour (grind organic rolled oats to flour)

¼ cup Quinoa flour (grind uncooked quinoa seeds in coffee grinder to flour consistency)

¼ cup rice flour or gluten-free baking mix

¾ teaspoon baking soda

1 teaspoon Italian seasoning

1/8 teaspoon salt (optional)

Wet Ingredients:

½ cup tofu

½ cup canned pumpkin puree or applesauce

2 teaspoons lemon juice

¼ cup almond butter or tahini

1 tablespoon olive oil

1 flax egg (see recipe index)

Method: Pre-heat oven to 350 degrees F. Sift dry ingredients into a large mixing bowl. Process wet ingredients in a food processor until smooth. Add wet ingredients to dry ingredients and mix well. Spoon batter into a 9 inch X 13 inch baking dish sprayed with olive oil. Bake 40 minutes. Test with a toothpick.

CHOCOLATE CHIP BLUEBERRY COOKIES

Dry Ingredients:

½ cup organic rolled oats (not quick oats)

½ cup oat flour

¼ teaspoon cinnamon

1/8 teaspoon salt (optional)

Wet Ingredients:

½ cup applesauce or canned pumpkin puree

2 tablespoons date syrup (see recipe index)

1 tablespoon olive oil

½ cup blueberries (fresh or frozen) *

½ cup plant-based chocolate chips.

Method: Pre-heat oven to 350 degrees F

Mix above ingredients in a medium mixing bowl until a sticky dough forms. Drop by heaping tablespoon onto a non-stick parchment paper lined baking sheet. Flatten with the back of a spoon to 2½ inch diameter. Bake at 350 degrees F for 30 minutes. Yields 12 cookies. Cool 10 minutes to set up.

Special notes: You are right…there is no leavening in this cookie. *Acceptable to substitute any small diced fruit for blueberries.

SWEET POTOATO SCONES

Dry Ingredients:

1 cup oat flour (grind oats in a coffee grinder)

¼ cup organic rolled oats

¼ cup rice flour or gluten-free baking mix (Kroger's brand)

½ teaspoon baking powder

½ teaspoon baking soda

½ teaspoon salt (optional)

Wet Ingredients:

1 cup cooked &peeled sweet potato, pureed

2 tablespoons almond butter or tahini

1 tablespoon olive oil

1 flax egg (see recipe index)

Method: Pre-heat oven to 375 degrees F.

Sift dry ingredients into a large mixing bowl. Combine wet ingredients in a medium mixing bowl. Add wet ingredients to dry ingredients. Stir to blend well. Drop batter by tablespoon onto a non-stick parchment paper lined baking sheet. Flatten scone to ½ inch. Bake at 375 degrees F for 20 minutes. When chilled, scones can be cut in half horizontally and filled with any spread or be a closed cucumber sandwich.

STRAWBERRY RICE CAKE TREATS

1 package unsalted rice cakes (health food store)

Strawberry jam (or any jam you like)*

Method: Spread jam on a rice cake for a sweet treat.

***No cook strawberry jam:** 1 pound of strawberries, about 20), cleaned, hulled and mashed, or any fruit you like. 2 tablespoons lemon juice. 2 tablespoons ground chia seeds (grind chia seeds in a coffee grinder). 10 drops of liquid stevia or 2 tablespoons 100% maple syrup. Combine ingredients in a large mixing bowl. Allow 2 hours for jam to set. Keep refrigerated.

Apricot-orange jam: ¼ cup orange date syrup (see recipe index) + ¼ cup jarred apricot jam. Mix in a small bowl. Keep in refrigerator up to 3 days.

Special notes about flour: Add 1/3 cup cornstarch to 3 cups of flour to make *cake flour.* The cornstarch lightens the flour.

Buckwheat flour is gluten-free. It is a seed (not grown as a grass). It is wheat-free, as well as a rich source of fiber and minerals. It is low to medium on the glycemic index and should not cause unhealthy spikes in blood sugar levels. Buckwheat flour is a complete protein. *Readers Digest.*

Note: Buckwheat flour can overwhelm a recipe. Add ¼ cup as a substitute for 1/4 rice flour and see if you like the taste. Works best with chocolate cake.

OATMEAL CAKE-LIKE SCONES

Dry ingredients:

½ cup oat flour (grind rolled oats to a flour)

1/3 cup organic rolled oats + ½ cup to sprinkle

1/8 cup rice flour

½ teaspoon baking powder

¼ teaspoon baking soda + a pinch of salt

Wet Ingredients:

2 tablespoons of date syrup or maple syrup

2 tablespoons olive oil

1/3 cup plant-based yogurt

¼ cup applesauce

¼ cup blueberries or any fruit (small dice)

Method: Pre-heat oven to 350 degrees F.

Sift dry ingredients into a medium mixing bowl. Mix wet ingredients in a separate medium mixing bowl. Add dry ingredients to wet ingredients. Mix well. Spoon dough onto a non-stick parchment paper lined baking sheet. Sprinkle batter with rolled oats. Wearing a disposable plastic glove, pat dough to an 8 inch circle. Score deeply with a knife into 8 wedges. Bake at 350 degrees F for 25 minutes. Test with a toothpick.

CHOCOLATE OATMEAL CAKE

Dry Ingredients:

½ cup organic rolled oats

½ cup oat flour (grind rolled oats to a flour)

¼ cup rice flour or gluten free baking mix

¼ cup cocoa powder

1½ teaspoons baking powder

¼ teaspoon salt

½ cup plant-based chocolate chips

Wet Ingredients:

½ cup applesauce

2 tablespoons olive oil

1 flax egg (see recipe index)

½ cup almond milk

1 teaspoon vanilla extract

4 tablespoons date syrup (see recipe index)

½ cup blueberries (fresh or frozen) or any small diced fruit you like or grated zucchini or grated carrots

Method: Pre-heat oven to 350 degrees F.

Sift dry ingredients into a medium mixing bowl. Mix wet ingredients in a small mixing bowl. Add wet ingredients to dry ingredients and mix well. Spoon batter into a Bundt pan or 9 inch X 9 inch baking dish, sprayed with olive oil. Bake at 350 degrees F for 35 minutes, until a toothpick inserted in the middle comes out clean. Cool in the pan 10 minutes.

To Serve: Frost with *Chocolate frosting*: one 6 ounce container of plant-based vanilla yogurt + one tablespoon 100% maple syrup or (date syrup-see recipe index) + one tablespoon cocoa powder. Mix ingredients in a small bowl until creamy. Keep in refrigerator up to 3 days.

To make *chocolate frosting* using sweet potatoes: Mash 1 cooked, peeled sweet potato (orange, garnet or gold sweet potato) with 2 tablespoons cocoa powder and 1 tablespoon 100% maple syrup or date syrup. Mash with a potato masher until smooth. Keep in refrigerator up to 3 days.

Health benefits of sweet potatoes: They are a great source of fiber, vitamins and minerals. Supports healthy vision. May enhance brain function. May support immune system (antioxidants). May have cancer-fighting properties. They contain beta-carotene and potassium. Sweet potatoes are a super food with a sweet taste. They are low on the glycemic index, which has less effect on blood sugar levels.

www.Healthline.com

DATE CAKE

Dry Ingredients:

½ cup oat flour (see recipe index)

¼ cup rice flour or gluten free baking mix

Wet Ingredients:

4 large pitted dates (½ cup), cut in half

½ teaspoon vanilla extract

¾ teaspoon baking soda

¼ teaspoon salt

½ cup applesauce

2 tablespoons olive oil

1 flax egg (see recipe index)

2 tablespoons date syrup (see recipe index)

Method: Process above ingredients in a food processor and let sit 15 minutes. Add dry ingredients and process until smooth.

Method: Pre-heat oven to 350 degrees F.

Pour batter into a 9 inch X 9 inch baking dish, sprayed with olive oil. Bake at 350 degrees F for 25 minutes until a toothpick inserted in the middle comes out clean. Yields 16 squares. Makes a tender cake.

Top with jam of choice.

<u>SO SOFT CHOCOLATE CHIP COOKIES</u>

Dry Ingredients:

¾ cup organic rolled oats (leave as whole oats)

¼ cup oat flour (grind rolled oats to a flour)

¾ teaspoon baking soda

1/8 teaspoon salt

½ cup plant-based chocolate chips

Wet Ingredients:

1/3 cup date syrup (see recipe index)

1/3 cup almond butter

Method: Pre-heat oven to 350 degrees F.

Sift dry ingredients (except chocolate chips) into a medium mixing bowl. Stir in chocolate chips. In a small mixing bowl, combine wet ingredients. Stir well. Add wet ingredients to dry ingredients. Stir well. Drop by teaspoon onto a non-stick parchment paper* lined baking sheet. Flatten slightly with the back of a spoon. Bake at 350 degrees F for 11 minutes. Cool 15 minutes on baking sheet. Yields 14 cookies.

*Reynolds Kitchens Cookie Baking Sheets are non-stick parchment paper. May need to order from internet if not in your grocery store.

MATCHA GREEN TEA COOKIES OR CAKE

Dry Ingredients:

½ cup oat flour (grind rolled oats to flour)

¼ cup rice flour or gluten free baking mix*

½ cup organic rolled oats (+1/4 cup for sprinkling)

½ teaspoon baking powder

¼ teaspoon baking soda

1/8 teaspoon salt (optional)

1 packet Matcha green tea powder

¼ teaspoon each cinnamon, cardamom** and vanilla bean seeds

Wet Ingredients:

¼ cup applesauce or Lekvar (pureed prunes)

2 tablespoons olive oil

2 tablespoons date syrup or 100% maple syrup

1 flax egg (see recipe index)

2 tablespoons almond milk

Optional add-ins: ½ cup chocolate chips or Craisins

*Kroger's brand:

** Maximum cardamom to add to any baking recipe is 1 teaspoon; more, gives recipe a soapy taste.

For cookies:

Method: Pre-heat oven to 350 degrees F

Sift dry ingredients into a medium bowl. Mix wet ingredients in a small bowl. Add dry ingredients to wet ingredients. Add stir-ins. Mix well. This is a wet, sticky dough. Drop by tablespoon onto a non-stick parchment paper lined baking sheet. Sprinkle each cookie with rolled oats and slightly flatten. Bake at 350 degrees F for 22 minutes.

For cake:

Method: Pre-heat oven to 350 degrees F

Combine and mix ingredients as above. Spray an 8 inch X 8 inch baking dish with olive oil. Pour batter into baking dish. Sprinkle with rolled oats. Bake at 350 degrees F for 25 minutes until a toothpick inserted in the middle comes out clean.

Serve topped with jam or cooked fruit.

Health benefits of matcha green tea powder: Packed with antioxidants. Boosts metabolism. Calms the mind and relaxes the body. Rich in fiber, chlorophyll and vitamins. Enhances mood and aids in concentration. Protects the liver. May help prevent cancer. Protects the heart. Helps with weight loss. *www. Healthline.com*

SUGAR-FREE FRUIT FUDGE

½ cup sugar free chocolate chips (Lilly's brand) or one sugar-free chocolate bar 2 ounce (Lilly's brand)

¼ cup applesauce**

1 tablespoon cocoa powder

1 tablespoon unsweetened plant based yogurt

10 drops of liquid stevia

1/8 teaspoon vanilla bean seeds

Method:

In a small microwave-safe mixing bowl, microwave the chocolate chips or chocolate bar and applesauce (high setting) 30 seconds. Stir. Microwave 30 seconds more, until chocolate is melted. Stir well. Add cocoa powder, yogurt, stevia and vanilla beans seeds. Stir well. Pour chocolate mixture into a 5 inch X 5 inch X 1 inch dish, lined with plastic wrap with ends of plastic wrap extending outside the dish by 2 inches. This will allow you to lift the fudge out of the dish. Chill in refrigerator 2 hours until set. Lift fudge out of dish and transfer to a cutting board. Cut into 16 one inch squares. Yields 16 servings. Keep refrigerated 3 days.

**Substitute: Sugar-free jam, or pureed cooked root vegetables (carrots, pumpkin or sweet potatoes).

Health benefits of oats: Rich in antioxidants. One of the healthiest grains. The soluble fiber in oats can lower cholesterol and improve blood sugar. Oats are a gluten-free whole grain. May reduces risk of heart disease. A good source of carbohydrates and fiber. Oats are the most nutrient dense food you can eat. ½ cup is 300 calories; 51 grams of carbohydrates; 13 grams protein; 5 grams fat; 8 grams fiber. Oats contain manganese, phosphorus, magnesium, copper, iron, zinc, folate, vitamin B1 (thiamin), vitamin B5 (pantothenic acid), calcium, potassium and vitamin B3 (niacin). Oats are rich in antioxidants and polyphenols. They can lower blood pressure by increasing production of nitric oxide. Oats are anti-inflammatory and promote good bacteria in the digestive tract. wwwhealthline.com

Recipe Index

D

E

F

G

H

I

J

Jams (see strawberry-orange, strawberry no cook, Blueberry, no cook, apricot, apricot-orange jam).

K

L

M

Index

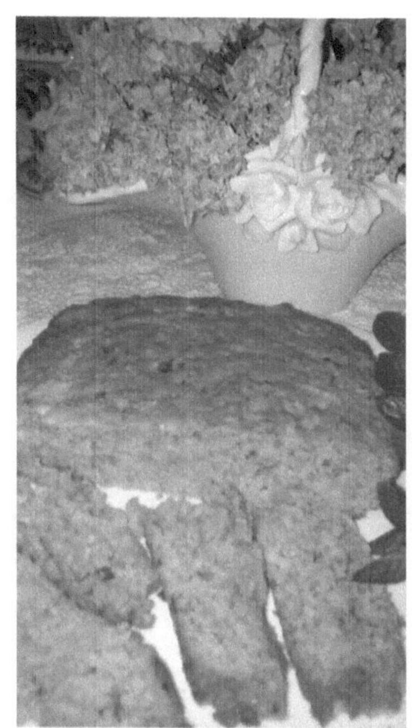

No yeast Bread

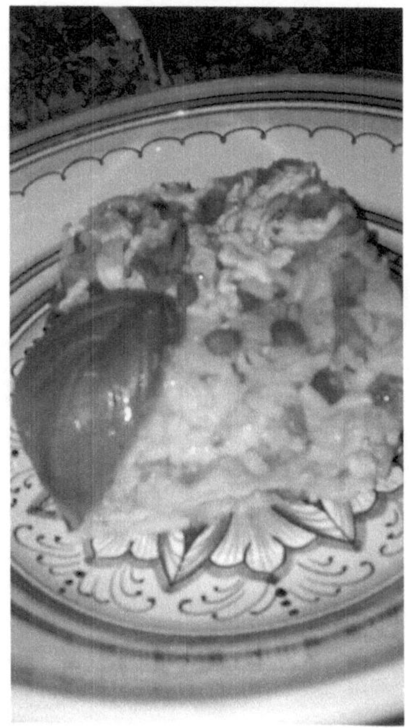

Green Chili Enchiladas

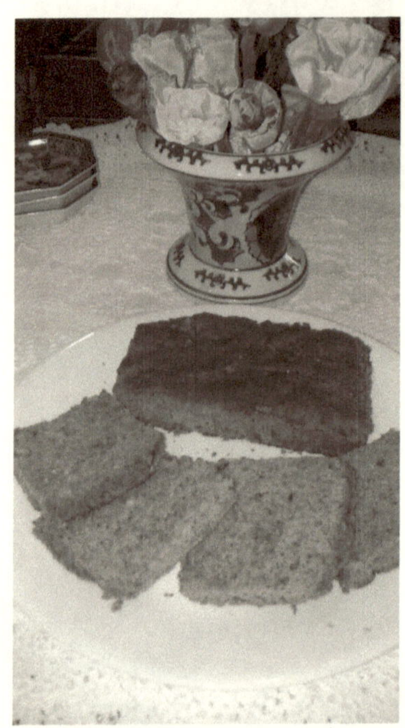

Zucchini Bread

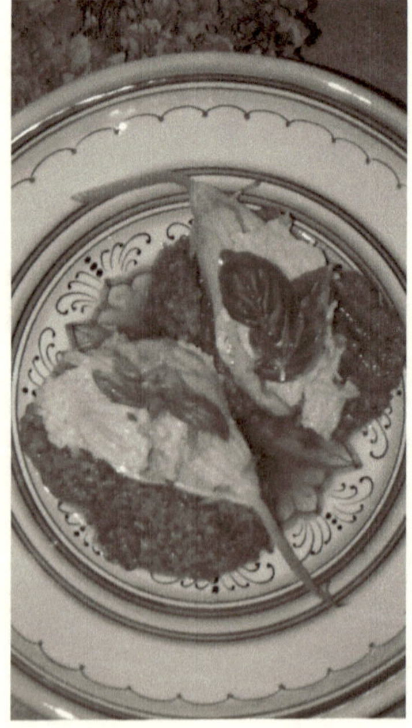

Baked Zucchini Flowers

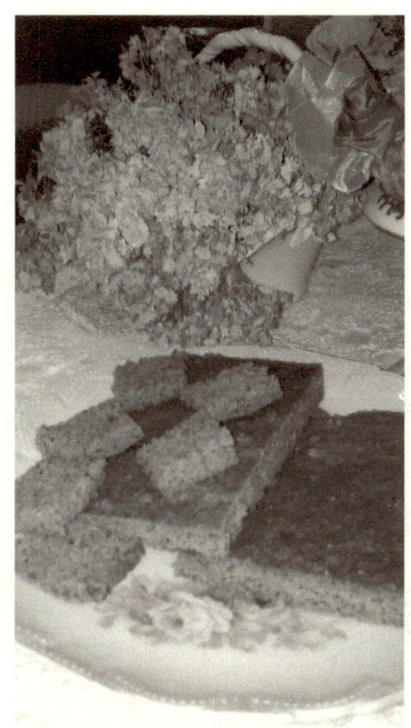

Tofu Ricotta Bread

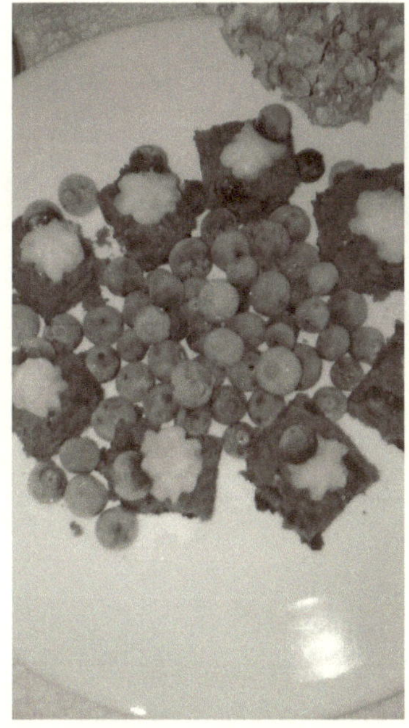

Citrus Cake with Blueberries

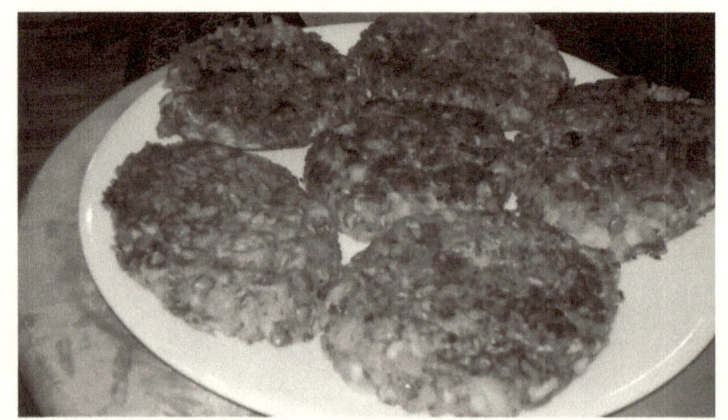

Bean Burgers

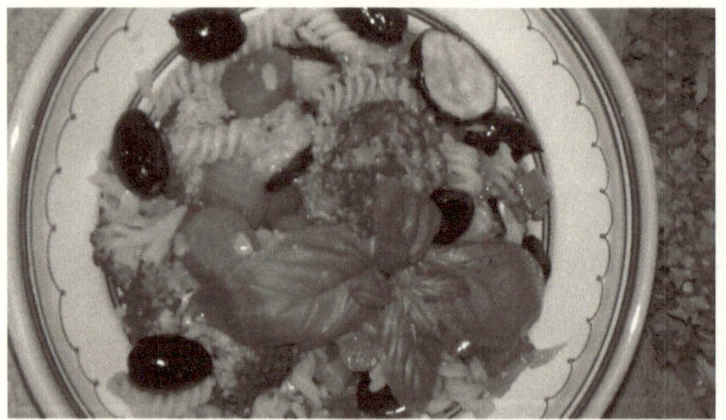

Pasta Salad

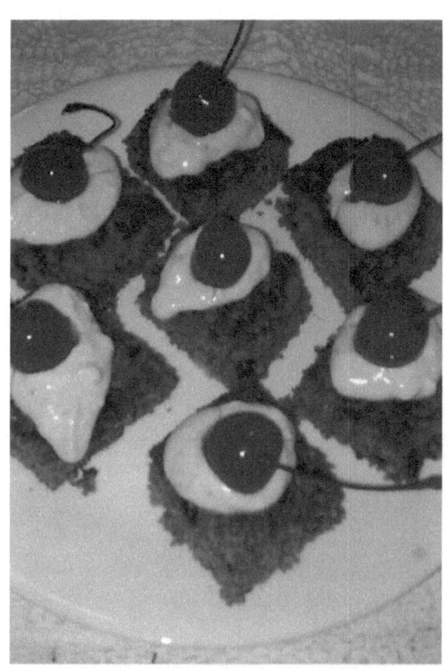

Carrot Cake with cherries

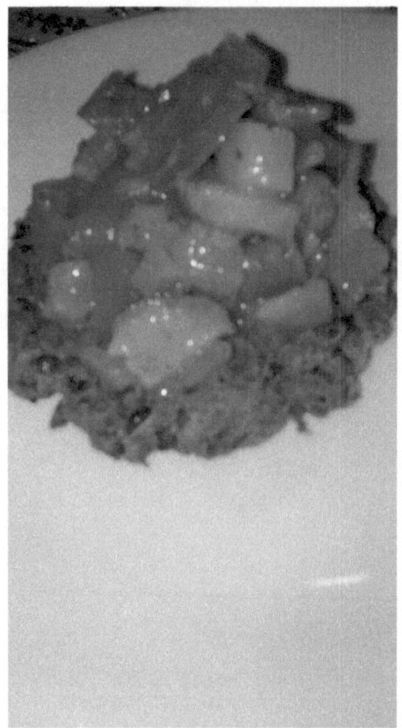

Vegie Burger with
Sweet and Spicy Pears

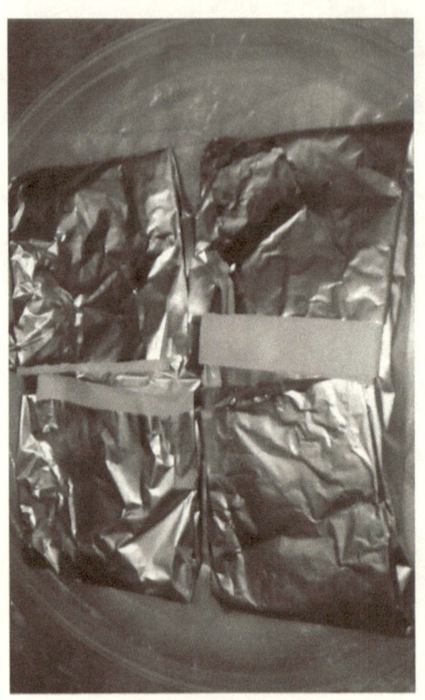

Tin foil Tamales

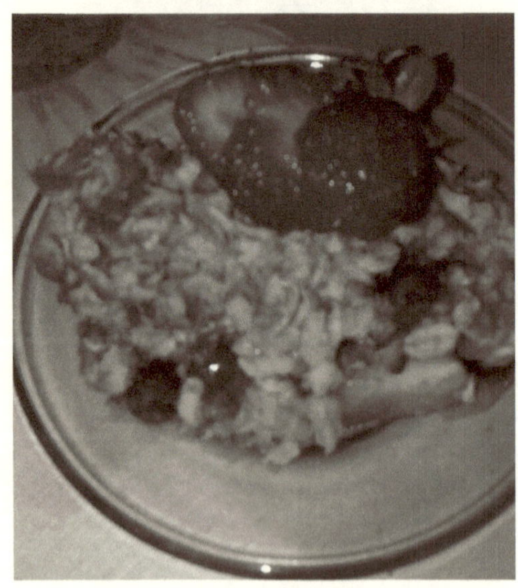

Baked Fruit

About the Author

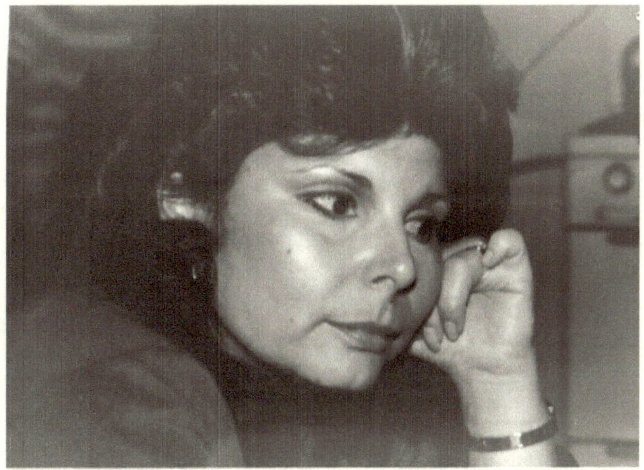

The author is an experienced Plant-based chef and teaches classes in Plant-based cooking. Other books by the author: Enlightened High Tea Parties. To view recipe pictures and new recipes see

www.vegansuperfoodrecipes.com